DESIGN OF LONG-TERM CARE FACILITIES

DESIGN OF LONG-TERM CARE FACILITIES

Laszlo Aranyi
Larry L. Goldman

VNR VAN NOSTRAND REINHOLD COMPANY

NEW YORK   CINCINNATI   ATLANTA   DALLAS   SAN FRANCISCO
LONDON   TORONTO   MELBOURNE

Van Nostrand Reinhold Company Regional Offices:
New York   Cincinnati   Atlanta   Dallas   San Francisco

Van Nostrand Reinhold Company International Offices:
London   Toronto   Melbourne

SB Copyright © 1980 by Litton Educational Publishing, Inc.

Library of Congress Catalog Card Number: 79-9567
ISBN : 0-442-26120-9

Manufactured in the United States of America

Published by Van Nostrand Reinhold Company
135 West 50th Street, New York, N.Y. 10020

Published simultaneously in Canada by Van Nostrand Reinhold Ltd.

15 14 13 12 11 10 9 8 7 6 5 4 3 2 1

Library of Congress Cataloging in Publication Data

Aranyi, Laszlo.
   Design of long-term care facilities.

   Bibliography: p. 207.
   Includes index.
   1. Nursing homes—Planning.   2. Nursing homes—
Design and construction.   3. Extended care facilities—
Design and construction.   I. Goldman, Larry L., joint
author.   II. Title.
RA997.A73   725'.56   79-9567
ISBN 0-442-26120-9

Foreword

As an administrator of a nursing home or long term care facility, I have become aware of a great diversity in our field. Homes vary in their size, and irrespective of their size, in the complexity of their organization: Sponsorship may be under proprietary or not-for-profit auspices; those operated for profit can have the administrator as the owner and sole developer. Some may be one home operations, others may involve partnership, and still others may be small, local corporations. Some proprietary sponsors can be large corporations, operating multi-facility chains on a regional or national basis. The non-profits can be similarly organized in complexity and oganizational sophistication, whether operated by religious, governmental or fraternal organization.

There is considerable pluralism in function, program and design because of ownership and management diversity. Accordingly, there may appear to be more dissimilarity than similarity between homes. However, if we accept as a premise that nursing homes by and large care for older people, we would assume that people with similar needs should be similarly sheltered. This assumption would also support the notion that there would be an accessible source of knowledge that would allow potential sponsors to make rational decisions in their own planning process. To the contrary, the authors found that the information was not easily accessible and what was available did not clearly identify its special relationship to caring for older people. Nursing home design seemed so patterned after health care facilities, such as hospitals, that their specialty in dealing with the needs of older people was not easily identifiable, if at all available.

The authors, in an attempt to design a nursing home, were not permitted to copy what already existed, unless they understood the special design conditions that related to the special needs of the aged. Instead, they were asked to experience, through simulation, the sensory deficits that comprise the life style of the older person. They were asked to examine environments in which the healthy aged and frail elderly live; to observe how they negotiate their environment and with what trepidation and tenuousness the aged person suffers an existence in an environment that is alien to his capabilities. In this effort, they become aware that the older person needing institutionalization moves from an external community to an internal community. He is more dependent both emotionally and physically in the institutional environment; the environment must therefore provide for as much compensatory assistance and stimulation as possible, in order to make the aged resident as functionally independent as possible. What follows, therefore, is an attempt to categorize in some way the considerations that must be taken into account when planning these environments. No attempt is made to suggest the "rightness" of their judgments, but there is a suggestion that each element of the total institutional community should be approached in a systematic fashion. They believe that their system is helpful, and I would concur. Most assuredly, they offer options in reviewing and planning which we believe are novel.

Ira C. Robbins, ACSW
Administrator
Beth Sholom Home of Virginia

V

Preface

The authors, an architect and an operator of long-term care facilities, were asked to serve as the project architect and a committee member, respectively, for a group seeking to develop a non-profit, long-term care facility. A search of the literature proved immensely disappointing, for little was written specifically for designers. There is a great deal written by, and for, social scientists and environmental psychologists, but the translation into architectural terms leaves a lot to be desired. The authors educated themselves by visiting a great number of facilities considered innovative and responsive to the residents' needs. Additionally, much time was spent interviewing residents, administrators and department heads of long-term care facilities, as well as architects. Notes became voluminous, giving birth to the idea of this book.

The subject of long-term care facilities is a complex one, and it is impossible to cover all aspects in one book. We hope this book will be of interest, help and encouragement to architects, interior designers, operators of long-term care facilities, governmental authorities and would-be sponsors of long-term care facilities. Hopefully, past mistakes in design would not be repeated and new ideas will be generated, resulting in a more humanistic housing for our aged population.

Laszlo Aranyi
Larry L. Goldman

Acknowledgments

Many people, including residents of long-term care facilities, contributed in many ways to this book. The authors are particularly indebted to William L. Freed, AIA, whose input regarding general design considerations and the format of this book was invaluable. Steven G. Roberts, P.E., and Herbert L. Sullivan, P.E., of Old Dominion Engineering supplied nearly all the material on climate control, plumbing, lighting and electrical design. Dr. Jan W. Abernathie provided all the technical material regarding the greenhouse, which is unique in that its design specifications must meet the needs of wheelchair-bound residents. Ms. Teresa Goldman, M.A., speech pathologist, provided the technical material for the section on a speech therapy room.

A very special thanks is due Ira C. Robbins, ACSW, Director of Beth Sholom Home, Richmond, Virginia, and his staff, as well as Ms. Mary Weathersby, Social Worker, and Ms. Barbara Gatewood, Activity Director, both of Health Care Center of Raleigh, Raleigh, North Carolina. These people read and criticized various parts of the text which, in the end, will make the long-term care facility more livable. Finally, credit is due Ms. Josephine D. Clark and Ms. Joan Keith, typists, who struggled with poor handwriting and many revisions in order to produce this text.

Contents

DESIGN OF LONG-TERM CARE FACILITIES

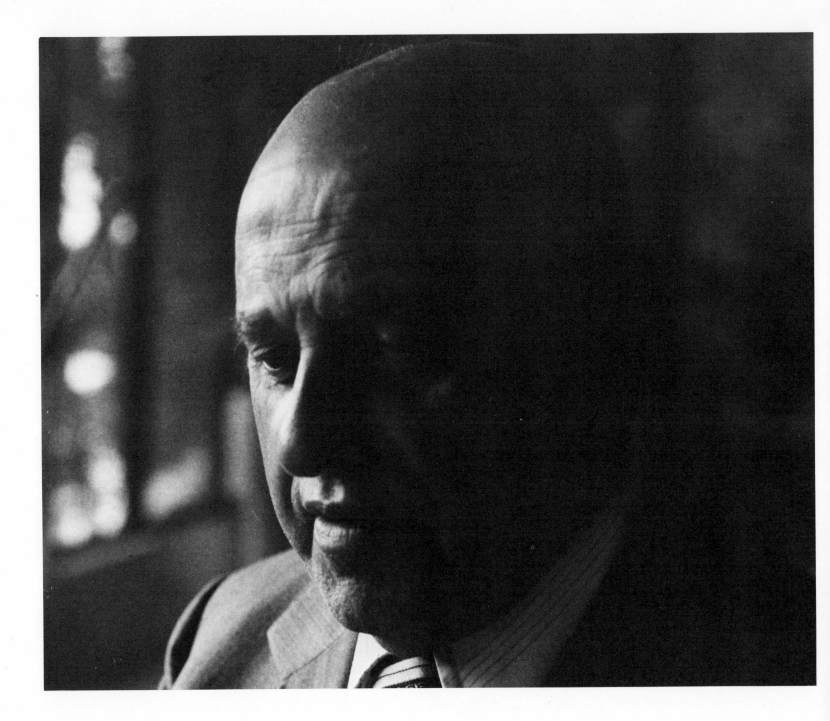

1.
Introduction

BRIEF HISTORY

Our attitude that care for the ill-aged should be provided by institutions has roots going back to sixteenth century England. It was then that responsibility for caring for the aged and infirm shifted from the church to the cities and towns. Almshouses sprang up in colonial America, although primary responsibility for the aged remained within families. Into the twentieth century almhouses, or county poor houses, continued to provide shelter for the aged. Living conditions were often wretched. In fact, so bad was the care and environment that the original Social Security Act, passed in 1935, specifically barred payment of assistance to the elderly housed in public institutions. Private institutions began to provide housing for the elderly and later many added a nurse; such facilities became known as nursing homes.

At the beginning of this century, there were only three million people (4% of the population) 65 years of age or older. With the advances in medical care, people began to live longer, life expectancy rising from 47 years in 1900 to better than 71 years presently. Our nation began a gradual shift from a largely rural to largely urban society and with this urbanization came smaller housing units and the need for greater mobility to follow factory work. Finally, Social Security decreased financial dependency of our aging population. The sum of these factors was the destruction of the extended family. In the meantime, the population aged 65 years or older reached 12.3 million in 1950 or 8.2% of the population.

The demand for facilities to care for the ill-aged began increasing in the 1950s, but significant growth did not develop until the enactment of Medicare and Medicaid laws in 1965. Health, Education and Welfare (HEW) statistics reveal that available nursing home beds increased from just over 500,000 in 1963 to over 760,000 four years later. The fact that the Federal Government contributed substantially to the growth of the nursing home industry is undeniable.

POPULATION TRENDS

The U. S. Census Bureau data published in 1972 graphically illustrates expected growth in the 65 years and older category.

U.S. POPULATION OVER AGE 65
1900-2000

Year	Total Population	Population Over Age 65 and Percentage of Total Population
1900	75,994,575	3,083,939 (4.1%)
1910	91,972,266	3,953,945 (4.3%)
1920	105,716,620	4,939,737 (4.7%)
1930	122,775,046	6,644,378 (5.4%)
1940	131,669,275	9,036,329 (6.9%)
1950	150,697,361	12,294,698 (8.2%)
1960	178,464,236	16,559,580 (9.3%)
1970	203,165,699	20,049,592 (9.9%)
1980	222,043,000	24,005,000 (10.8%)
1990	238,910,000	27,566,000 (11.5%)
2000	251,056,000	28,337,000 (11.3%)

Source: U.S. Bureau of the Census. *Population Estimates and Projections*, Series P-25, Number 493, December 1972, p. 26.

The U.S. Department of Health, Education and Welfare, in 1975, published its projection that by the year 2000 there will be 31 million elderly 65 and over—60% of them women. It should be noted here that while women always outnumber men by a small percentage, in long-term care facilities women outnumber men three to one.

As could be expected this population is not evenly distributed across the nation. In fact, 35% of the nation's aged crowd into five states—New York, California, Pennsylvania, Florida and Illinois; the

1

same states account for 33% of all the nation's population. Not surprisingly, over 15% of Florida's population is 65 years of age or older compared to just over 10% in the nation as a whole. While Florida houses 3.7% of the nation's population, it is home for 5.6% of the 65 years and older population segment; this is, however, the only sunbelt state where the population mix significantly favors the aged.

NEW TRENDS IN CARING FOR THE AGED

The application of the knowledge of the problems of the aged to the construction of long-term care facilities is the purpose of this book. A body of knowledge is being developed with respect to these problems, but the solutions to these problems architecturally are slow in coming. It would be useful for the designer and the developer to spend a day in a long-term care facility, confined to wheelchairs and wearing eye glasses made translucent by the application of petroleum jelly to the lenses. Surely then a more humanistic design would be the result.

Long-term care facilities are still being designed using the hospital as a model. The result is a facility with a strong institutional image. The aged population which must be housed in long-term care facilities for health reasons has a need for a particular social-psychological atmosphere.

Where Long-Term Care Facilities Fail

Typically, an aged person who yesterday decided what time he would wake up, what he would eat for breakfast and what he would wear is thrust into a new and unfamiliar environment where all of those decisions are made for him. He is robbed of his independence; his self-esteem begins to suffer; he becomes disinterested in himself and begins to require increasing amounts of care. The staff encourages this dependence, because they get impatient with the speed at which a resident dresses himself or answers a question. This is a major failing of most long-term care facilities.

Humanizing Factors

The negative impact on the resident produced by this dependence is not the only problem thus created: Dependence also increases the need for staff. Long-term care facility leaders were slow to recognize the problem and even slower in devising effective responses. In all

fairness, it must also be understood that many residents upon admission have already been made dependent by well-meaning family members.

Restoration of some degree of independence is being accomplished by assuring that vision, hearing and speech defects are being corrected where possible, and that mobility is maintained through the use of therapy or aids to ambulation. Currently, leaders are beginning to deal with the problem from the social-psychological aspect in some interesting ways. Some facilities have "General Stores" where various articles of clothing, toiletries, etc., are sold. The clothing might be used and priced very inexpensively, but the resident has an opportunity to make his own selections. He must also pay for these items with his own funds. A facility in New York serves buffet style. While some residents complained about standing in line, the overwhelming response has been that of gratitude for the opportunity to express a preference. This method of food service does not result in significantly higher food cost. In order to assure the resident of getting his choice of foods, two or three meat dishes and two to four vegetable dishes are prepared. After the residents have eaten the staff will eat what is left over. An Activity Director who is well trained and strongly motivated can develop a crafts program which will result in the production of saleable items. It is recommended that residents participating in the program share in the "Profits" equally. Nothing builds a sense of self-worth faster than to earn pay for work done. Some states stupidly discourage this kind of activity by reducing financial assistance to the resident by the amount of money he earns in this fashion.

The Overall Plan of Care

All states now emphasize the resident's "overall plan of care." There was a time when the plan of care was nothing more than a medical-nursing plan. Today, the plan might include elements from the physical therapist, the activity director, the social worker, the dietition and direct care workers (aides/orderlies).

Reality Orientation

Increasing emphasis is also being placed on reality orientation. Because of the diminution of the senses and for other reasons, many residents begin to display symptoms usually labeled as senility. It has been found that this condition can be markedly improved if the resident is constantly reminded of who he is, where he is, what day it is, what season it is, etc. This is called reality orientation and requires the total involvement of all the staff from housekeeping to administrative personnel. Reality orientation ought to be an on-going staff development program.

Elsewhere in the text there will be other thoughts dealing with architectural considerations as they pertain to resident care.

GLOSSARY OF TERMS

AIDE: A nurse's assistant.

CERTIFICATE OF NEED: States require that a sponsor of a nursing home must prove that the need for those beds exists. Such a certificate is issued for a limited period of time, usually a year, and can be extended provided progress has been made.

DIETITIAN: A person who has a baccalaureate degree and has completed an internship approved by the American Dietetic Association, or who has equivalent education and training.

FIRE DOOR: A fire-resistive door assembly, including the hardware, which under standard test conditions, meets the fire protective requirements for the location in which it is to be used.

GERIATRICS: A branch of medicine dealing with the problems and diseases of the aged.

INCONTINENCE: Involuntary loss of urine and/or feces.

INTERDISCIPLINARY TEAM: A team composed of representatives from the following disciplines from within a facility: nursing, social services, activities, medical, dietary and sometimes physical therapy, occupational therapy and even housekeeping. The team is responsible for assessing the resident's needs and devising and monitoring the plan to meet those needs.

INTERMEDIATE CARE FACILITY (ICF): A nursing home differing from a skilled facility, in that it offers a lower level of nursing care but otherwise is likely to be identical in physical plant. The ICF resident differs from the rest home resident, in that he will have several medical problems, may require treatments, injections, etc.

LONG-TERM CARE: Services for symptomatic treatment, maintenance, and rehabilitative services for residents of all age groups in various health care settings.

MEDICAID: Title XIX of the Social Security Act was enacted in 1965 and provides for grants to states for medical assistance programs. It is a joint program of the federal and state governments, designed to provide medical care for persons, irrespective of age, who would otherwise not be able to pay for such care.

MEDICARE: Title XVIII of the Social Security Act became effective 1965, and provides for hospital and post-hospital care for persons 65 years of age or older.

NURSING HOME: A facility which is licensed by the state to provide nursing care. The state has standards relating to the physical plant, care, services, staffing, etc. which must be met in order for the facility to be licensed; also called long-term care or extended-care facility.

ORDERLY: The male counterpart of the aide.

PRIVATE PATIENT: A resident who pays for his own care, as opposed to a Medicaid or Medicare patient.

PROPRIETARY FACILITY: A facility operated for profit.

REALITY ORIENTATION: A process by which disoriented persons are helped to be less confused. Any worker from whatever discipline who is likely to come in contact with the confused resident participates in the process by reminding the resident of: his name, where he is, the hour, day, or season of the year. Most facilities have several reality orientation boards scattered throughout the facility. See "Graphics and Signage" for further discussion.

RESPONSIBLE PARTY: Refers to a person who is financially responsible in whole or in part for a resident.

REST HOME: Like the nursing home these are also licensed by the state pursuant to well defined standards. They provide a lower level of care, usually catering to persons requiring no nursing services; also called home for adults. The resident of such a facility is up and around and is usually able to perform the activities of daily living, such as grooming, dressing, feeding, etc.

SKILLED NURSING FACILITY (SNF): The highest level of nursing care available in nursing homes. The SNF resident differs from the ICF resident, in that he will require extensive medical and nursing care, may be bedridden, may have indwelling catheters, may be tube fed, etc.

THIRD PARTY PAYOR: An insurance company or agency of the state or federal government that pays for the care of a resident.

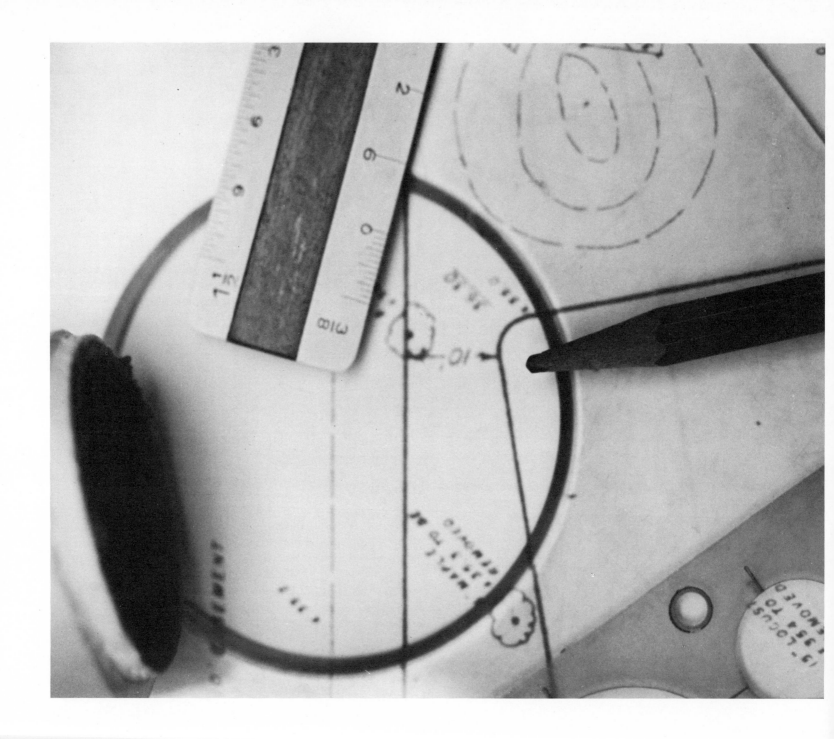

2.
Getting Started

THE FIRST STEPS

Unless you already know your way around in the long-term care business, getting a project like this started can be so frustrating that abandonment becomes a serious consideration. The following are agencies or people whose counsel should be sought at the beginning of the project in order to keep it viable:

1. The State Health Department is usually the licensing and regulating authority within the state. There are likely to be several people in the department with whom you should meet: start with the head of the department and quickly outline your project for him. Be candid and do not try to hide your ignorance; make friends.

2. The State Department of Welfare (or Social Services or whatever department it is that manages Medicaid) should be your next stop. The State, through the Medicaid program, has become the largest purchaser of long-term care services. Like the State Health Department, the Medicaid agency will also have a list of standards which must be met, in order for a facility to be allowed to participate in the program. Again, be candid. It would be foolhardy for a proprietary facility to open its doors without Medicaid certification for the reason that 70 to 80% of long-term care residents are Medicaid recipients.

3. The agency responsible for Comprehensive Health Planning must be consulted at an early stage. This organization has the responsibility of determining if you have proved the need for your proposed facility. Without their approval, it will be impossible to get Medicaid certification.

4. Visit someone already in the business. This might well be the first person you should visit. A friend already in the field can save lots of time and useless effort; don't be timid, most are willing to help.

5. An architect who has designed and built nursing homes in the state in which the proposed facility is to be located can be of immense assistance. Ask to see some facilities of his design which have been built, and also find out what they cost to build.

6. See a mortgage lender or broker. If money is generally available for mortgages, but not for nursing homes in your state, then proceed cautiously. He would be able to give you tentative mortgage terms, so that a probable debt service could be calculated. You will need to know this for inclusion in your pro forma operating statement, an example of which is shown elsewhere.

7. An attorney should be consulted to determine what legal structure the facility should take. Usually a corporation is best for a variety of reasons; this is not the time to incorporate, however. Much will have to be accomplished first to be certain that the project has a reasonable chance of getting off the ground.

SITE SELECTION

One might be tempted to select some bit of pastoral acreage for a long-term care facility. This might be appropriate for horses but not for people. Long-term care residents want to see activity, especially human acitivity, and such activity is even more stimulating when it is not associated with the facility. In general terms, a good site will be one in a residential area, with perhaps some commercial area nearby, and where there are some community activities that would encourage the resident to leave the facility for short times and participate; such activities might be cultural, religious, or sporting events.

Other important considerations:

- Availability of public transportation
- Availability of utilities (sewer, water, storm drainage)
- Availability of proper zoning
- Availability of restaurants for the convenience of staff

- Absence of site problems:
  Poor drainage
  Bad topography
  Poor soil bearing characteristics
  Difficult accessibility
  Potential hazards to safety
  Close to noxious odors
  Close to noise
- Adequate size for the property to accommodate the building, parking, outdoor recreation and possible future expansion

SELECTION OF CONSULTANTS

The consultants' work will be more beneficial when they are involved from the inception of the project; it must be noted that a consultant can only advise. The decisions will have to be made by the governing body or the business entity. An experienced consultant can be of immense help in avoiding or overcoming problems. The selection of consultants is a vital part of the overall planning process and very similar to hiring an employee but a great deal more critical. The selection should be done in a systematic manner, which includes the following basic steps:

- Invitation to a number of firms to submit the following information:
  experience
  qualifications
  specialized abilities
  resumés of key personnel
  present work load
  services offered
- Evaluation of the submissions to determine which firms are the best qualified. The evaluation should be based on the following:
  performance on previous assignments
  familiarity with the type of project at hand
  professional standing of key people
  expressed interest in this project
  familiarity with local codes, standards and procedures
  references
- Interviewing the representatives of the highest ranking firms to narrow the field down to the most qualified. The interviewing process should explore in depth the items listed under 'invitation' and 'evaluation.'

- Ranking of the top three firms based on the personal interview.
- Fee negotiation with the top ranking firms. Consulting fees are generally based on staff time, plus expenses, such as travel, telephone, printing, computer time etc. Fees will range widely according to the amount of staff time and expertise required and the reputation of the firm. Whatever the arrangement is, it should be put in writing to avoid conflicts later on through misunderstanding.

Attorney

Very often the first consultant to be selected is the attorney. His role will be many-faceted and will generally include legal work in the following areas:

Formation of sponsoring agency or business entity
Identifying legal regulatory constraints
Land acquisition and transfer of title
Reviewing contracts with other consultants
Assisting in obtaining zoning approvals
Assisting in obtaining Certificate of Need
Reviewing construction contracts
Reviewing permanent and construction financing documents

Architect

More than likely the second person or firm to be selected will be the architect. This consultant should be employed even before a site is selected. Some of the work will be done by the architect in-house, or he may employ a consultant himself when it comes to some specialty with which he is not familiar. Generally, the architect can provide professional services in the following areas:

Existing facilities survey (in case of an alteration job)
Economic feasibility
Site selection
Preliminary engineering report
Programming
Preliminary cost estimates
Zoning approvals
Master planning
Certificate of Need
Federal, state and local agency approvals

Graphic material for fund raising
Building design
Interior design
Landscape design
Contract documents
Bidding or negotiating with contractors
Observation of construction
Approval of payments to contractors
Post construction services

Interior Designer

If the architect does not provide this service, a separate firm will have to be employed. The interior designer should work very closely with the architect. The interior designer can provide the following professional services:

Preliminary furniture layout to assist the architect in determining room sizes
Selection of interior wall, floor and ceiling finishes
Color coordination
Final furniture and equipment selection
Selection of window treatment products
Selection of accessories (lamps, clocks, interior greenery, etc.)

Accountants

There are accounting firms with special knowledge regarding long-term care facilities. Such a firm could provide professional services from the inception of the project in the following areas:

Feasibility studies
Certificate of Need
Tax counseling
Bond counseling
Pro forma statements
Financing

Construction Manager

In the last few years a new breed of consultants has emerged to replace the old bidding method of awarding the general construction contract. Traditionally, the low bidder will get the job, and, very often, the entire construction time is spent negotiating over various items which the general contractor feels should be an "extra," while the architect and the owner strongly resist. The construction management process will eliminate a lot of these problems, because the construction manager works directly for the owner for a fee, and consequently he has no direct financial interest in the total construction cost, except to keep it as low as possible. He is part of the team; services provided include:

Consulting with the architect during the preparation of construction documents
Preliminary cost estimating
Evaluation of alternate construction methods and building products
Final cost estimate
Taking sub-bids
Negotiating with sub-contractors
Managing construction

Miscellaneous Other Consultants

Space does not permit going into further detail, but there are many other consultants who could be retained on a limited basis. Some of these will be used even after the facility is in operation:

Kitchen designer
Consulting dietitian
Pharmacist
Social worker
Management consultant
Security consultant
Programming
Gerontologist
Medical services consultant
Graphics consultant
Public relations consultant
Fund raiser
Market analyst

References:

Directory of Consultants for the Development of Facilities for the Aging:

> American Association of Homes for the Aging
> 2050 Seventeenth Street, N. W.
> Washington, D. C. 20036

How to Find, Evaluate, Select, Negotiate with an Architect:

> The American Institute of Architects
> 1735 New York Avenue, N. W.
> Washington, D. C. 20006

CODE INFLUENCES

The long-term care facility will have to conform to a great number of codes and regulations, in addition to the usual building and fire prevention codes. The following is a list to alert the designer to check out all the relevant ones. One word of caution: Some of the codes may have conflicting requirements. Additionally, in most states the completed construction documents will have to be approved by the State Health Department or similar agency.

- Local and/or state building codes
- Local and/or state fire codes
- State Health Department requirements for long-term care facilities
- HUD minimum property standards
- National Fire Protection Association
  Life Safety Code—NFPA 101
- H. E. W. Interpretive Guidelines and Survey Procedures for the Application of Standards for the General Intermediate Care Facilities:

  > 45 CFR 249.12 (a) and (b)
  > September 3, 1974
  > Published by: American Health Care Association
  >   1200 15th Street, N. W.
  >   Washington, D. C. 20005

- Minimum Requirements of Construction and Equipment for Hospital and Medical Facilities:
  > DHEW Publication No. (HRA) 76-4000

8

FINANCING

Long-term care facilities are financed in the traditional ways: i.e., banks, savings and loan institutions, insurance companies and by a not-so-traditional route—Industrial Revenue Bonds. The developer will usually approach the bank or savings and loan in his community directly; however, loans from insurance companies are most often arranged through mortgage brokers. Financing via Industrial Revenue Bonds requires the services of a bond specialist. This method frequently results in very satisfactory financing but is not permitted in every state. The bond specialist will be able to quickly advise regarding state law.

The Mortgage Package

The mortgage package usually contains the following:

> Pro Forma Operating Statement
> Preliminary Site Development Plan
> Preliminary Floor Plan of the Building
> Outline Specifications
> Personal and/or Corporate Financial Statements of the Developer

The Pro Forma Operating Statement. The developer must concern himself with preparing the pro forma. Most lenders are sophisticated and informed, or they will seek an opinion from an expert in the field of financing long-term care facilities. The pro forma must be reasonable and complete if the developer is to obtain financing.

Developing a monthly pro forma operating statement, when taken a step at a time, is not a terribly difficult task. What follows is the construction of a pro forma statement for a 120-bed intermediate care facility based on the staffing requirements of a Mid-Atlantic state. Cost data are developed first, since Medicaid income will be tied to cost. Costs will be frequently expressed in terms of "cost per patient per day" or "cost per patient day."

The format.

> Income:
>
> > Medicare
> > Medicare Co-Insurance
> > Private
> > Medicaid

Medicaid Co-Insurance
Veterans Administration
Meal Sales (i.e. to visitors)
Vending Machine Income
Resident Laundry
Barber/Beauty Shop
Medical Supplies
  Total Income

Expense:

Administrative Department:

Administrator
Office Salaries
Fringe Benefits
Supplies
Repairs and Maintenance (i.e. Typewriters, Business Machines)
Administrative Expense (a catch all)
State Unemployment Tax
Federal Unemployment Tax
FICA Tax
Equipment Rental (i.e. Office Machines, Automobile)
Travel
Training and Education
Dues and Subscriptions
Casual Labor
Insurance, General
Insurance, Workman's Compensation
Telephone
Legal
Accounting
Utilities
Interest Expense
Advertising
Licenses
Property Taxes
Postage
Freight
Trash Disposal
Management Fee (commonly charged in chain operations)
  Total Administrative Expense

Nursing Department:

Salary: Director
Salaries: RN's
Salaries: LPN's
Salaries: Aides/Orderlies
Salaries: Therapists
Salaries: Activity Workers
Salaries: Social Workers
Fringe Benefits
Medical/Nursing Supplies
Clerical Supplies
Repairs and Maintenance
State Unemployment Tax
Federal Unemployment Tax
FICA Tax
Equipment Rental
Travel
Training and Education
Insurance, Workman's Compensation
Non-Legend Drugs
Laboratory Fees
Utilization Review
Social/Activities Supplies
Therapy Supplies
Medical Director
Professional Services (i.e. Consultants)
  Total Nursing Department Expense

Dietary Department:

Dietary Salaries
Fringe Benefits
Supplies (i.e. Paper Products, Cleaning Chemicals)
Repairs and Maintenance
State Unemployment Tax
Federal Unemployment Tax
FICA Tax
Equipment Rental
Travel
Training and Education
Insurance, Workman's Compensation
Raw Food
China, Glassware and Silver
  Total Dietary Expense

Housekeeping Department:

Housekeeping Salaries
Fringe Benefits
Supplies
Repairs and Maintenance
State Unemployment Tax
Federal Unemployment Tax
FICA Tax
Equipment Rental
Travel
Training and Education
Insurance, Workman's Compensation
Total Housekeeping Expense

Maintenance Department:

Maintenance Salaries
Fringe Benefits
Supplies
Repairs and Maintenance (i.e., Independent Contractors)
State Unemployment Tax
Federal Unemployment Tax
FICA Tax
Equipment Rental
Travel
Training and Education
Insurance, Workman's Compensation
Total Maintenance Expense

Laundry Department:

Laundry Salaries
Fringe Benefits
Supplies
Repairs and Maintenance
State Unemployment Tax
Federal Unemployment Tax
FICA Tax
Equipment Rental
Travel
Training and Education .
Insurance, Workman's Compensation
Linens
Total Laundry Expense

Non-Controllable Expense:

Building Rent (if appropriate)
Depreciation
Total Non-Controllable Expense

Other Expense:

Federal Income Taxes
State Income Taxes
Local Income Taxes
Total Other Expense
Total All Expense
Total Net Income (Loss)

The format is very detailed, and if the purpose is to obtain financing, it may be simplified by combining many line items within a cost center giving a total dietary cost, for example.

Most of the cost centers in our example contain common line items such as:

Fringe Benefits
Repairs and Maintenance
State Unemployment Tax
Federal Unemployment Tax
FICA Tax
Uniform Expense
Rental Equipment (not included elsewhere)
Travel
Training and Education
Workman's Compensation Insurance

The above line items, as another alternative, may be combined to give a total for say "fringe benefits," irrespective of the cost center.

Fleshing it Out. Since the number of beds available in a state is rigidly controlled, it is fairly safe to predict a 94% occupancy, which will be attained after the initial fill-up period (about a year). Therefore, patient days will be 3429 (120 beds x 30.4 days x .94) for a month. A special note must be interjected at this point. The primary purpose of this pro forma is to obtain financing. *It cannot be used as a budget without further refinement.* Months do not have 30.4 days, they have 28 days, 30 days and 31 days, and the difference can be significant: Consider the difference in income between a 31-day month and February. The difference in patient days will be

120 beds x 3 x .94 = 338.4. The income loss will be then 338.4 patient days x $30 (a typical ICF Medicaid rate in the Mid-Atlantic states)—$10,152. Many expenses, but not all would be scaled down accordingly. It is a trap which must be avoided.

In the income of our pro forma, we have assumed that 80% of the residents are beneficiaries of the Medicaid Program and that the state rate for Medicaid is cost plus $1.50 profit per patient day. It can be seen readily that the cost of Medicaid care was $73,214 ($91,518 total cost x 80%) and Medicaid patient days were 2743 (3429 patient days x 80%). Therefore, the Medicaid rate for our facility was $28.19 ($73,214 Medicaid cost ÷ 2743 Medicaid days = $26.69 plus $1.50 for allowable profit equals $28.19) and Medicaid income becomes $77,325 ($28.19 Medicaid rate x 2743 Medicaid days) which is the same as the sum of the Medicaid and ''Medicaid: Resident Portion'' line items on the pro forma.

Starting with ''Administrative Department,'' the process begins by considering one line item at a time. The *Administrator* will ordinarily command an annual salary of $10,000 to $20,000. We will use $1,500 per month. We expect to need three *office workers*: one bookkeeper, one secretary-bookkeeper and one secretary-receptionist. Inquire as to the usual wage for each skill in the community. Making wage projections is the wrong place for guessing. For example, we may have selected as the site for this facility the medical center of a three county area; however, that very fact is likely to mean keen competition for health care workers. Prevailing wages indicate filling these three positions will cost $1,548/month.

The *other administrative expenses* used in the illustration were derived from actual costs (1978). The insurance expense is for comprehensive coverage. Workman's compensation varies widely from state to state and local state law should be consulted. ''Utilities'' expense is an average, so again be careful, because this cost will vary considerably with the season and with geographic location.

The *Nursing Department* expense is largely in labor cost. The state has set up minimum staffing requirements for the nursing department, an example of which follows. Nursing labor cost projections become a matter of pricing out the staffing required by the state or better by the condition of the residents for whom the facility is being constructed.

CENSUS	DAY NUMBER NURSING PERSONNEL	EVENING NUMBER NURSING PERSONNEL	NIGHT NUMBER NURSING PERSONNEL
41- 50	3-4	3-4	1-2
51- 60	4	4	2-3
61- 70	5	5	2-3
71- 80	5-6	5-6	2-3
81- 90	6	6	2-3
91-100	6-7	6-7	2-3
101-110	7	7	3
111-120	8	8	3
121-130	8-9	8-9	3
131-140	9	9	3
141-150	10	10	3

For more than 150 residents a ratio of 1:15 for the first two shifts and 1:30 for the night shift are considered minimums; these minimums include nurses as well as aides and orderlies (A/0). This state requires one nurse only on the day shift for each 100 residents or fraction thereof, 8 hours per day, 7 days a week. One of those nurses is to be designated as nursing supervisor; however, the state also requires that a facility be staffed to meet the needs of the residents. Experience indicates that our proposed facility would need at least two nurses on each of the first two shifts and one on the night shift and aides/orderlies would likewise have to be increased. Additionally, a director of nursing will be necessary; therefore, a reasonable staffing for this proposed facility would be:

	DAY	EVENING	NIGHT	TOTAL
Aides/Orderlies	10	9	6	25
Nurses	2	2	1	5

All nursing staff is to be under the supervision of the Director of Nursing.

To complete our cost projections, all that need be done now is to finish the calculation.

25 aides/orderlies x 30.4 days x 8 hours x hourly rate = Total Wages: A/O

5 nurses x 30.4 days x 8 hours x hourly rate = Total Wages: Nurses

The Director of Nursing will earn usually between $11,000 and $15,000 annually

This same process will be used to determine labor costs in each of the other departments. Other nursing expenses are typical.

The *Dietary Department expenses* are for a facility employing conventional means of preparing, serving and storing foods. Since all states require that no more than 14 hours shall elapse between a substantial evening meal and breakfast, the hours of dietary workers are likely to vary from other facility workers. Most facilities serve the heaviest meal around noon, so staffing will be greatest around that time. One 125-bed facility uses the following schedule:

HOURS	COOKS	DIETARY AIDES
6:00 A.M.—2:30 P.M.	1	2-3
10:30 A.M.—7:00 P.M.	1	1
2:00 P.M.—7:00 P.M.		2-3

Additionally, this facility employs one worker in the kitchen who does the heavy cleaning and the maintenance. All of these workers are managed by the dietary supervisor. After labor cost, the next most significant cost is for raw food. In our example we chose $2.00 per patient day as the likely food cost. This cost multiplied by 3429 (the patient days determined earlier) will give an estimated monthly food cost of $6858.

The *Housekeeping Department* and *Laundry Department* are frequently managed by the same person. In both departments, labor is the major cost. About 960 hours of labor per month would be required in housekeeping for this 120-bed facility, while the laundry would require about 450 hours. Housekeeping supplies will cost on the average $700 per month, and laundry supplies will cost $550 to $650 per month.

The *Maintenance Department's* major cost is labor, just as is every other department's. Maintenance employees will be required to work approximately 226 hours each month.

Finally, there are the categories of expenses labelled in our illustration *"Non-Controllable"* and *"Income Tax"* which are self-explanatory.

Using the above information we can now fill in the numbers. Some of the figures used were arrived at by the process just described. The other figures were taken from financial reports of facilities operating in a Mid-Atlantic state and may be considered typical for the region and for 1978.

The finished product.

Monthly pro forma operating statement

Income:

Medicare	—0—
Medicare Co-Insurance	—0—
Private	$20,367
Medicaid	66,490
Medicaid: Resident Portion	10,835
Veterans Administration	—0—
Meal Sales	140
Vending Machine Income	50
Resident Laundry	840
Beauty/Barber Shop	—0—
Medical Supplies	—0—
Total Income	$98,722

Expense:

Administrative Department:

Administrator	$1,500
Office Salaries	1,548
Fringe Benefits	384
Supplies	333
Repairs and Maintenance	25
Administrative Expense	100
State Unemployment Tax	70
Federal Unemployment Tax	19
FICA Tax	210
Equipment Rental	510

Travel	417
Training and Education	50
Dues and Subscriptions	16
Casual Labor	24
Insurance: General	600
Insurance: Workman's Compensation	20
Telephone	360
Legal	50
Accounting	1,000
Utilities	2,813
Interest Expense	100
Advertising	70
Licenses	5
Property Tax	2,070
Postage	70
Freight	26
Trash Disposal	44
Management Fee	6,500
Total Administrative Expense	$18,934

Nursing Department:

Salary: Director	$ 1,125
Salaries: RN's	2,030
Salaries: LPN's	3,300
Salaries: Aides/Orderlies	18,370
Salaries: Therapists	1,130
Salaries: Activity Workers	1,000
Salaries: Social Workers	1,000
Fringe Benefits	—0—
Medical/Nursing Supplies	2,000
Clerical Supplies	85
Repairs and Maintenance	—0—
State Unemployment Tax	710
Federal Unemployment Tax	190
FICA Tax	1,770
Equipment Rental	—0—
Travel	5
Training and Education	40
Insurance: Workman's Compensation	175
Non-Legend Drugs	150
Laboratory Fees	—0—

Utilization Review	150
Social/Activities Supplies	240
Therapy Supplies	27
Medical Director	450
Professional Services	—0—
Total Nursing Department Expense	$33,947

Dietary Department:

Dietary Salaries	$5,925
Fringe Benefits	—0—
Supplies	700
Repairs and Maintenance	160
State Unemployment Tax	126
Federal Unemployment Tax	34
FICA Tax	353
Equipment Rental	16
Travel	—0—
Training and Education	—0—
Insurance: Workman's Compensation	34
Raw Food	6,858
China, Glassware, Silver	90
Total Dietary Expense	$14,296

Housekeeping Department:

Housekeeping Salaries	$3,200
Fringe Benefits	—0—
Supplies	700
Repairs and Maintenance	5
State Unemployment Tax	86
Federal Unemployment Tax	22
FICA Tax	204
Equipment Rental	—0—
Travel	—0—
Training and Education	5
Insurance: Workman's Compensation	240
Total Housekeeping Expense	$4,462

Maintenance Department:

Maintenance Salaries	$1,100
Fringe Benefits	—0—
Supplies	450

Repairs and Maintenance	300	
State Unemployment Tax	28	
Federal Unemployment Tax	7	
FICA Tax	70	
Equipment Rental	5	
Travel	—0—	
Training and Education	—0—	
Insurance: Workman's Compensation	7	
Total Maintenance Expense		$1,967

Laundry Department:

Laundry Salaries	$1,030	
Fringe Benefits	—0—	
Supplies	650	
Repairs and Maintenance	12	
State Unemployment Tax	13	
Federal Unemployment Tax	3	
FICA Tax	30	
Equipment Rental	—0—	
Travel	—0—	
Training and Education	—0—	
Insurance: Workman's Compensation	3	
Linens	35	
Total Laundry Expense		$1,776

Non-Controllable Expense:

Building Rent	$14,400	
Depreciation	1,736	
Total Non-Controllable Expense		$16,136

Other Expense:

Federal Income Taxes	*		
State Income Taxes	*		
Local Income Taxes	*		
Total Other Expense		*	
Total All Expenses (except "Other Expense")		$91,518	
Total Net Income (Loss)			$7,204

    * No attempt is made to determine taxes due

This pro forma was developed out of years of experience and up-to-the minute cost and income information. An understanding of the State's Medicaid Program is essential in preparing the income portion of the pro forma. Many state Medicaid programs limit profit severely or provide for no profit at all, and typically Medicaid residents would make up about 70% to 80% of the resident population. Question other local long-term care facilities about the rates private residents are paying, in order to get an idea of what rates are possible. There are facilities that are 100% private, but there are more facilities that are 100% Medicaid. It is important to be prudent in planning at this stage; a great deal of money will be at risk.

That experience counts is beyond question. Engaging experienced people to head departments can insure the financial success of the venture. The operation of long-term care facilities is often times described as as a "Pennies" business. This is true, and, for this reason, the administrator who is long on experience is an insurance policy against financial disaster. Likewise, strength in nursing and dietary is essential. For reasons other than strictly financial, an experienced activity director will add the dimension of humanness: love, caring, warmth and stimulation.

Floor Plan, Outline Specifications and Site Plan. The architect will supply the floor plan, site plan and the outline specifications. The architect should not proceed beyond this stage until financing is secured.

Financial Statements. The lender will almost always insist on the personal and/or corporate financial statements of the project's developer. Likely, too, will be the requirement of the personal endorsement of the developer. Knowing this at the outset should emphasize the necessity of preparing a thoughtful pro forma.

LICENSING

The licensing procedure begins prior to commencement of construction. In fact, the licensing authorities will have to approve the plans, specifications and the site. During construction, representatives of the licensing authority will visit the site to ensure compliance with the plans and specifications, and occasionally they will make new requirements, which could be costly.

When the building is finished and furnished and all systems are working, the licensing authority will order a final inspection. This inspection is thorough and will include testing the fire alarm system, nurse-call system and checking the sprinkler system. If this final inspection is successful, the facility will be licensed to admit its first residents.

CERTIFICATE OF NEED

The developer will be required to apply for a "certificate of need." In other words, the developer must prove to the Health Planning Agency that the need for the proposed beds exists. Certificate of need forms are lengthy and detailed. Questions posed will be concerned with:

- The financial viability of the project
- The availability of both professional and non-professional workers
- The availability of public transportation
- Tentative cost of the site, building and furnishings
- The availability of residents

The answers to these questions and others must be supportable. Nothing can kill a project faster than making questionable statements on the certificate of need application. Reliable information will be obtained from various state agencies, chambers of commerce, local governments, the federal government, census reports etc. The certificate of need is a necessary step to satisfy the rules and regulations, but certainly the developer should want to satisfy himself that the project is needed.

The certificate once issued will carry with it an expiration date of usually one year. The agency provides for renewals of the certificate, if the developer can prove that he is making substantial progress. The certificate is issued for a particular site, plan, number of beds and to a particular developer, whether private or corporate. Changes are possible but must be approved by the agency.

Ordinarily, the agency is not a single entity but several agencies. Usually, there is a local body which limits its concerns to a certain geographical area. They will recommend to the state agency approval or disapproval of the project. The state agency can override a decision of the local body. The local organization is most often composed of a paid professional staff and state or local appointees from the community and supposedly representative of the community.

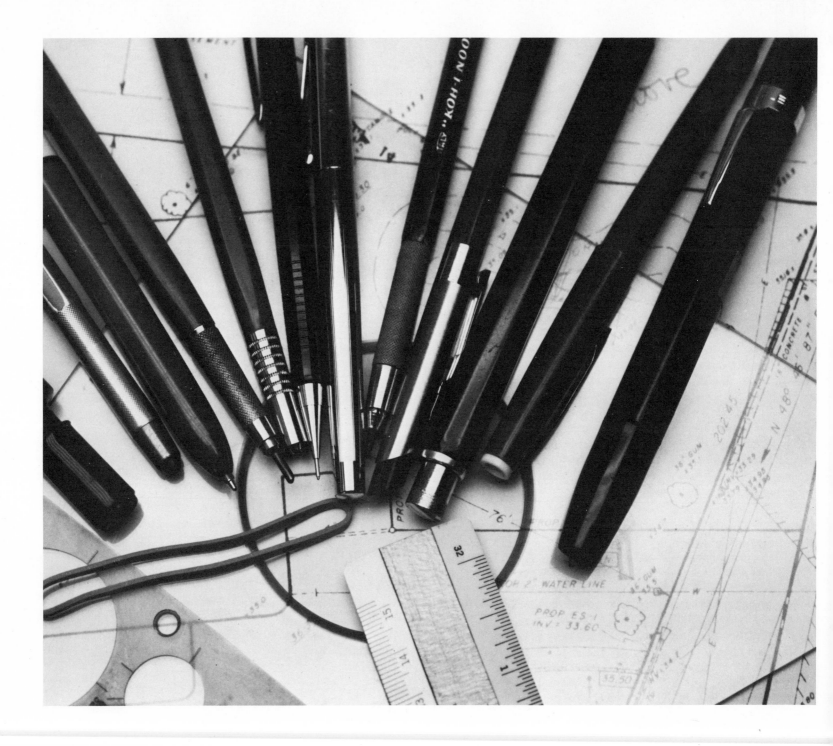

eeping it from being istitutional while still being functional.

3.
General Design Considerations

SPACE

Space is where things happen. The way space is enclosed, that is the size and shape, including the height of the room, plays an important part in the long-term care facility. The idea is that, in general, a space should have a singular, unambiguous definition and use. The purpose is to compensate the environmental arrangements for lessened sensory acuity. Space should be cued with landmarks which act as focal points for functionally different spaces. For example, color-coded surfaces can signal functionally different spaces in terms of visual perception, textured surfaces for the tactile sense, and so forth. The purpose is to sensorially load the spaces, so that they may more effectively serve as points of reference and avoid ambiguous messages. It should be kept firmly in mind that the changes in sensory acuity and other important psychological factors of this population are such that subtle and/or complex architectural solutions are not only unappreciated but are confusing.

Design Considerations

The optimal size of any space must be determined by the activity or activities which will take place in the area, the number of people who will be involved and the furniture, equipment and supplies which are needed. Even with this information, it is very difficult to give a definite prescription for the size required for any given area. We must also keep in mind that we are designing for individuals who may be confined to wheelchairs or have other handicaps and need large space in which to maneuver. The long-term care facility must be designed keeping in mind the people who will use it the most:

people to take into consideration

- Residents. They may spend many years of their lives there.
- Staff. The facility must have good working conditions for many different types of workers, some of whom will sometimes be performing unpleasant tasks.
- Volunteers. These people give freely of their time to help the aged and the sick.
- Visitors (family). Family members have guilt feelings about putting people in long-term care facilities. Pleasant surroundings will surely ease this burden.

The shape of the rooms should be such that easy, casual supervision is possible.

Scale

We should remember that large rooms with high ceilings have a very institutional feeling about them. Lower ceilings tend to create a more residential atmosphere.

Scale is the relationship between the human body and its environment. Before planning spaces and selecting furniture and equipment for the elderly, it is necessary to understand the characteristics of the aging process, and how the resident will function in the facility. Proper scale is achieved by giving consideration to such items as the interior proportions of space, the size and shape of furniture, equipment, fixtures, and the height of operating hardware, windows, railings, electrical switches, and the like. Scale can give a facility a residential or institutional atmosphere. Scale and form properly executed can produce an atmosphere of order and beauty. The size and shape of the space in a long-term care facility should receive careful consideration, because of the influence these factors have on the behavior and well-being of those who will use it.

people confined to wheel chairs

17

INTERIOR SURFACES

Interior surfaces are an important aspect of the environment in stimulating vision and the sense of touch. Interior surface materials should be selected after careful consideration of their hygienic qualities, color, light reflectance, acoustical qualities, textural qualities, insulation value, durability and initial and maintenance cost.

Walls

The walls of the long-term care facility are used for many things besides defining the rooms. The usage of the walls should be kept in mind when the surface material is selected. It should also be remembered that equipment placed on the walls should be kept below normal height, because a great number of the residents may be confined to wheelchairs and elderly people in general are shorter. This is true of windowsills, as well as tack boards, signs and other communication media. There should be a variety of wall treatment in a long-term care facility: smooth, rough, soft, and hard.

Walls and doors should be easily and inexpensively maintainable, especially the parts that are within reach. Glossy surfaces should not be used in order to avoid glare. Vinyl wall covering is an excellent material in areas that require frequent cleaning.

Floors

Floor materials should be chosen with such characteristics as: smoothness, ease of maintenance, warmth, resilience and water resistance; other factors, such as wheelchair and walker maneuverability should be considered. The floor material may also be considered for its acoustical properties. Experience has proven that carpet in long-term care facilities in areas where some of the residents may be incontinent is a constant maintenance problem and therefore should be avoided. The problem with resilient flooring, besides having an institutional connotation, is the high reflectance, causing objectionable glare in the eyes of the elderly residents (glossy finish should be avoided completely). There is a definite need for the development of a new product to combine the low reflectance and soft appearance of carpet and the water resistance of resilient tile.

Ceilings

Ceilings may be more textured than walls and floors, because they do not come into direct physical contact with the occupants. Ceilings should be used mainly for sound distribution or absorbtion. There are various types of acoustical ceilings on the market, and it is suggested to use several types in the facility to differentiate between functions. The resident rooms should have the more residential-type, while the administrative and service spaces can use the regular, commercial types. Water resistance should be considered in areas where moisture will be present. Fire rating will be required in many instances, and the local codes must be consulted in this matter.

Other Surfaces

Other surfaces to be considered: built-in equipment and furniture, windows, doors, door frames, hardware, light fixtures, mechanical equipment, etc. Generally these should have a flat, non-glossy finish, with low light reflection.

COLOR

Carefully chosen color will not only contribute to the beauty of a long-term care facility, it will also create a beneficial psychological effect on the behavior of all who use the facility. There are general responses to color which are widely accepted. Many studies have led to interesting observations about color which are useful in understanding how color may affect the behavior of older people.

Most residents of long-term care facilities have opacity of the eye lens, which causes all colors to appear faded. The cool colors, such as green and blue fade most, while reds tend to fade the least. Another problem with elderly people is contouring, the capacity to perceive the boundary between two adjacent surfaces; this is most apparent when two intense colors such as red and green are next to each other.

There is evidence of increased activity, alertness in the presence of warm and luminous colors, thus creating an environment which is conducive to muscular effort, action, and cheerful feeling. As the following charts show, red produces tension, excitement, and a feeling of warmth, while blue results in a feeling of well-being. Color treatments

carpet makes it look more like home but you soaked is ① much worse

for elderly

COLOR	GENERAL PSYCHOLOGICAL RESPONSE
BLUE	peaceful comfortable contemplative restful
BLACK	despondent ominous powerful strong
WHITE	cool pure clean
YELLOW	cheerful inspiring vital
PURPLE	dignified mournful
RED	stimulating hot active happy
ORANGE	lively energetic exuberant
GREEN	calm serene quiet refreshing
PASTEL COLORS	neutral non-respondent soothing

should be based on the use of the room, as well as the length of time it will be used. The size of the surface area to be colored should be considered: large surfaces should be in pastel and soft hues, while small surface areas should be strong, bright colors.

Contrary to what might be expected, there is reason to believe that some excitable individuals respond more therapeutically to stimulating colors, and withdrawn individuals, to cool colors. In other words, some people respond best to colors which are in sympathy with their own emotional condition.

Doors in different colors can help the residents distinguish the closet from the hall or bathroom. Colors can also individualize residents' rooms, giving them a sense of territory. The color and texture of furniture should provide strong contrast to the floor. This will help many residents avoid bumping into furniture. Color-coding can also help the residents get about more easily; for instance, a colored stripe on the floor a foot from the wall helps in judging distances for wheelchairs and walkers. Handrails tend to be more obvious if painted brightly. The handrail and floor stripe can be the same color, and each separate residential wing can have a different color scheme. However, colors and patterns must be carefully selected to avoid optical confusion or dizziness.

In the selection of colors for long-term care facilities the anticipated responses must be considered, as well as the purpose for which the area will be used, the people using the area, the size of the space, natural light and other physical characteristics. Personal color preferences should also be considered in the resident rooms, since, in some instances, these are occupied for long periods of time by a single person.

DESIGN

Most facilities are designed for the resident's children, who must place them in such a facility, or for the convenience of the administrators and staff who will operate the facilities. The residents' rooms are usually set up for the convenience of the staff. Once the bed, table and chair are arranged, they are rarely moved from that spot, even though a small change might provide a better or different angle from which to view the outside world.

The following is an edited excerpt from a speech made by Otto Fuchs, Architect, New York State Department of Health in 1972:

One of the basic requirements in the design of a long-term care facility is to provide wheelchair users and other handicapped persons with access and ease of movement within the facility, both through the exterior and the interior spaces. The residents' use of equipment and conveniences, as well as their participation in all activities is another basic design consideration.

Perhaps we should think of a long-term care facility not simply as a building, but a total living environment containing aspects of physical, intellectual, and emotional past environments. A long-term care facility is also a place where persons come because of physical illness or age and spend all their time. A long-term care facility should, therefore, provide more than is found in an everyday home, because it replaces the street, the terrace, the park, the town, etc. The residents are greatly concerned with their immediate surroundings, because such surroundings are their total environment. The color of the walls, the shape of the walls, the shape of the rooms where they spend so much time—all these seem to be of greater importance to residents of a long-term care facility than they are to us in our daily lives.

The psychological and social needs of older adults must be considered in the design process. The following list of needs is from Lorraine Hiatt Snyder:

1. Maintenance of individual identities; the development of a positive concept of one's self.

2. Love; affectional physical contact.

3. Meaningful activity; creative activity; activity which is not busy work or "make" work.

4. The feeling of self-reliance; the sense of independence, perhaps through a reduction of environmental demands.

5. Stimulation; excitement of living; curiosity arousal.

6. A safe, dignified, efficient environment provides opportunity for both social interaction and privacy.

7. The opportunity and option of controlling or regulating one's own daily living; chance to control various aspects of one's physical setting, schedule, and activities.

8. The opportunity to keep track of time, to differentiate one day from another, to be oriented to temporal changes.

9. An opportunity to reflect on the past (termed life reviews) as a means of understanding one's self in preparation for the future.

ODOR CONTROL

Odor is a problem in every long-term care facility. Some facilities deal with it more successfully than others. Every facility is likely to have some incontinent residents; so why do some facilities smell better than others? The answer is complicated. First, odor is generally a nursing problem, because it is the aide or orderly who is summoned when a resident has an "accident." The aide/orderly must quickly change soiled clothes and linens and place the soiled items in a container with a lid. These items should never be first dropped on the floor nor should underpads, if they are used, be placed in the resident's trash receptacle.

The problem becomes a housekeeper's problem when the floor or furniture is also soiled. When that situation exists, the housekeeper should respond promptly. Frequently the problem is made worse by the housekeeper, who uses a single bucket, instead of a double bucket mopping system. Actually, when using a single bucket system, the housekeeper is spreading across the floor in his mop water the very cause of the odor rather than eliminating it.

Effective Mopping

In the double bucket system, the clean mop is dipped into the first bucket containing the cleaning solution and applied to the floor. The mop is then wrung out in the second bucket and dipped again into the first bucket with the cleaning solution, repeating the process until a manageable area has been swabbed. Next, the floor is mopped dry, the wet mop being wrung dry into bucket number two.

Selecting the Right Furnishings

Proper selection of furnishings will also go a long way toward eliminating this disagreeable problem. Mattresses should always have waterproof ticking. Seating used by residents should also be covered in materials that shed or repel liquids. If these rules are observed, there should be no need to use deodorants which themselves oftentimes have disagreeable odors. First and foremost, odor control is a nursing problem and a good director of nursing will see to it that such a problem does not exist.

Carpeting Not Recommended

Probably nothing creates residential atmosphere and adds warmth to a long-term care facility like carpeting, but carpeting soaked with the urine of incontinent residents gives off an odor so disagreeable that nothing justifies its use. According to statistics approximately 60% of the residents have bladder control difficulties. The standard solution has been to use vinyl asbestos tile, sheet vinyl, or terrazzo. The problem with all these is that they project an institutional quality.

SECURITY AND SAFETY

Actually security is a multifaceted problem; the security of the resident and his belongings being the major consideration; however, the security of the workers and their belongings and the security of the building and its furnishings must also be considered. Security really refers to freedom from danger and from fear. This means that there is a "feeling" component in the word security. Therefore, the problem has a psychological aspect. How do you promote a secure feeling among the people living and working in a long-term care facility? You give them reasons to feel secure, such as evidence of:

Fire Alarm Systems
Fire Extinguishers
Smoke Detectors
Sprinkler System
Panic Hardware on Doors

Drawers and Cabinets with
Locks for Personal Belongings
Lockers for Workers
Absence of Suspicious People
Security Guards

In December 1977, Institutional Management Magazine conducted a survey regarding security problems in various institutions and published the following results:

	HOTEL/ MOTEL	HEALTH CARE	COLLEGE/ UNIVERSITY	ELEMENTARY/ SECONDARY SCHOOL
Vandalism	30.9%	26.6%	25.8%	56.6%
Theft: internal	25.0	22.5	19.3	12.1
Theft: Break-ins	20.2	11.5	18.8	25.5
Drugs	4.8	12.4	9.3	8.5
Personal security	7.4	21.6	14.2	7.2
Fire: arson	7.4	12.0	10.2	9.0
Other	4.3	3.4	2.4	0.8

Courtesy of Institutional Management magazine

Access Control

Criminals can enter as visitors, maintenance or service personnel or other technical people. What complicates matters further is the fact that while a long-term care facility is in operation 24 hours a day, 7 days a week, the service and office areas are in operation only 8 to 10 hours a day and 5 days a week. When the service and office areas are closed down, only the nurses stations are attended, leaving the front entrance and service entrance often without surveillance. The presence of a security guard or a television monitoring system might be the answer, although this may affect some people adversely. Choice of neighborhood could obviate the need for a security guard or television monitoring system. The placement of the employee entrance near or in view of a nurses station, or any other place in the building where there are likely to be people at all hours, could eliminate the need for such security measures. If it is determined to use security guards, there are "contract" guard services available, and generally they are more economical than an in-house organizaton. A recent survey by *Institutional Management Magazine* found that in the health care field just over one fifth of the respondents used contract services. This was the highest percentage of all institutional groups. Television security monitors smack of big brotherism and are particularly offensive, with the possible exception of their use at the central supplies receiving point. Some facilities have very strict controls and even issue employee badges. Particularly in urban setting, the main entrance and the service entrance should be located in view of well travelled streets.

Protection of Personal Property

The residents should be provided a means of protecting their belongings. Since the rooms cannot be locked, they should have a drawer and/or cabinet equipped with locks. This introduces another problem, which is the loss of keys. Obviously, the need for master keys is essential. A duplicate set of keys should be kept in a safe place. Similarly, the workers need a secure place to lock up their outer clothing, pocketbooks, etc. (See Staff Locker Room)

Exit Control

Frequently, long-term care facilities have residents who must be protected from themselves. Every experienced long-term care facility administrator has tales to tell about residents walking out of the facility onto a busy street, down a ravine, falling into a river or the like. There was even one story about a resident who found a vacant automobile with its motor running, drove it down the street, and eventually wrecked it. The best safeguard against this potentially tragic problem is to always have plenty of staff about. And it's everybody's problem . . . nursing, housekeeping, etc. Alarms which sound when a door is opened work quite well during those hours when staff is minimum. There are also newer developments in hardware design, enabling the staff to lock or unlock the exit doors by remote control. This system must be connected to the smoke or fire alarm system, whereby the doors will automatically unlock in case of an emergency or power failure.

Protection of Equipment and Supplies

Thought must also be given to protecting the sizable investment in building and furnishings. Already cited were the fire safety features and the possible use of television monitoring. Additionally, the placement of entrances where traffic can be monitored readily by workers is of great value. Business machines, nursing, housekeeping and maintenance equipment when not attended should be locked up. Inventories and serial numbers of such equipment should be maintained in a safe place and reviewed often. There are many accountants today who are still depreciating items of equipment in long-term care facilities which are no longer at the facility because of having been stolen.

The security of drugs is well set out in each state's rules and regulations, and the reader is referred to them. However, it is important to note that the existence of drugs in a facility invites thieves both from the outside and from within.

Employee Screening

Many facilities have adopted a policy of making a condition of employment that a worker submit to polygraph tests if requested. Pre-employment screening should always include a check of references and police records. It is also a good idea to put workers on notice (in writing) that employees leaving work with bags or packages may be subject to a search of those parcels. Statistics show the majority of losses can be attributed to employee theft. Linen is particularly vulnerable to theft.

Inventory Control

Stringent inventory controls for drugs and linens are a must. In the orientation program new employees must be made aware that such controls are in existence and that employees caught stealing will be prosecuted.

Outdoor Lighting

It is very important to provide good lighting around the parking lots and exterior walks. This will help the night shift feel more comfortable entering or leaving the building.

Key Control

The number of keys and master keys must be carefully controlled and only authorized people may keep them. The architect and the administrator must carefully work out the keying system, and it might be advisable to have a hardware consultant present, who is familiar with the various codes. Many times the security requirements are in direct conflict with the code requirements.

Accident Prevention

Floors must be non-slip for the protection of the residents, as well as the employees. Most employee accidents occur in the food service and the laundry areas and are caused by spillage. In resident areas, glare (reflected light from the floors) must be avoided as much as possible. In the interest of the appearance of cleanliness, housekeeping workers tend to make floors very shiny, which in turn will temporarily blind old people with impaired eyesight.

Walls of very rough surface must be avoided to prevent accidental injury to residents, corners should be rounded for the same reason. Handrails are required in most areas where residents will be walking. Ends of handrails must be turned back to the wall for safety. According to statistics, over 90% of resident accidents involve falling. The place of these accidents were:

Bedroom	65%	Dayroom	6%
Bath	13%	Other	5%
Hall	11%		

Fire Safety

Even though a building is constructed out of fireproof materials, this fact does not eliminate fires. All buildings can burn and particularly the furnishings, draperies, and other contents. When administrators encourage residents to bring personal items, even furniture, from their home this increases the fire hazard. The first item to catch on fire is likely to be a piece of clothing or the bedding material when a person drops a cigarette on it. Then it spreads to the drapery, carpet, etc. The basic goal of fire protection is to limit combustible materials and then limit the spread of fire by compartmentation. Automatic sprinkler systems seem to provide the best protection and are a requirement in all new construction.

All new long-term care facilities are required to have smoke and fire alarm systems with audible and visible indicators. Regular fire drills are required by law, and the staff must be prepared to act fast and in an orderly manner in case of an emergency. State fire inspectors make regular visits to detect any violation or non-compliance. Fire extinguishers are generally required to be located in certain areas. The local fire department should be consulted in this matter.

BARRIER-FREE DESIGN

There is a strong movement to make all buildings accessible to the handicapped. It is particularly important for a long-term care facility to be made completely barrier-free, including employee areas. All 50 states in the United States have laws regarding barrier-free design. A lot of those simply refer to the standards for accessibility by the American National Standards Institute known as ANSI A117.1, currently under revision.

One of the earlier codes which provided excellent information was developed by the State of North Carolina and is still used by many professionals. The proliferation of state barrier-free codes has created a great deal of confusion. The designer must consult the local, state and federal codes having jurisdiction. The designer must also consider a lot of details beyond the ones listed in the guidebooks. The elderly have special problems with operating certain types of hardware or turning the conventional faucets. Leon A. Pastalan developed the "Empathic Model," which enables the designer to experience first-hand the problems related to aging. The Empathic Model consists of a series of appliances simulating the visual, auditory and tactile sensitivity of an aged person.

The following is a list of design information sources for barrier-free design:

1. An illustrated handbook in the Handicapped Section of the North Carolina State Building Code—North Carolina Department of Insurance, P. O. Box 26387, Raleigh, N. C. 27611
2. "The Disabled Need Not Be Handicapped" by Bradley Corporation, P. O. Box 309, Menomonee Falls, WI 53051
3. National Center for a Barrier-Free Environment, 7315 Wisconsin Ave. N.W., Washington, D. C. 20014
4. Architectural & Transportation Barriers Compliance Board, 330 C. St. S.W., Room 1010, Washington, D. C. 20201
5. President's Committee on Employment of the Handicapped, Committee on Barrier-Free Design, Washington, D. C. 20210
6. The National Easter Seal Society for Crippled Children & Adults, 2023 W. Ogden Ave., Chicago, Ill. 60612
7. Eastern Paralyzed Veterans Association, 432 Park Ave., South, New York, N. Y. 10016. This group publishes books explaining national barrier-free laws and state laws of New York, Pennsylvania, New Jersey and Connecticut.
8. Barrier-Free Site Design, U.S. Government Printing Office, Washington, D. C. 20402, Stock Number 023-000-00291-4

SINGLE STORY VS. MULTI-STORY BUILDINGS

There is no clear consensus as to which one is more desirable, when confronted with the question, "Do you prefer single-story or multi-story building?" Invariably, the preference expressed by the administrator was for the building he was currently managing. In other words, the administrator of a single-story facility would build the same kind of building again, and the administrator of a multi-story building would opt for the multi-story version. If there is sufficient land available at a reasonable cost a one-story building should be built. However, in an urban setting the long-term care facility will end up being a multi-story building due to high land cost.

Single-Story Building

Advantages:
- Easy evacuation
- Closeness to nature
- Permits residents to go outside more readily
- Simple traffic pattern
- Lower construction cost

Disadvantages:
- Long corridors
- Takes up a lot of land space
- Less security

Multi-Story

Advantages:
- Uses less land area
- Fireproof construction
- Residents may feel more secure

Disadvantages:
- Elevators required
- Transportation of residents becomes difficult
- Residents prefer to be close to the ground
- Difficult evacuation process, particularly if elevators are out of commission
- Food service is more complicated, because of the possible need to transport food to dining rooms on various levels
- Higher construction cost

FURNISHINGS

The main thrust of this guidebook is to encourage the creation of an environment which promotes a feeling of well-being, of independence, of individual worth, and an atmosphere which engenders the continued growth of the resident. All that effort would be wasted by unimaginative selection of furnishings. Resident furnishings must be of sufficient variety to appeal to different tastes and must always be residential looking.

Most manufacturers of resident-room-furnishings are able to meet both the need for residential appearance and nursing convenience.

Residents should be allowed, even encouraged, to individualize their rooms, and this means that some residents will bring in pieces of furniture, creating the need for a storage area for the displaced furnishings. In multi-bedded rooms great care must be taken in selection of room furnishings that will allow for "territoriality." The resident must know and feel that this is "my bed, my chest, my chair," etc. This can be achieved through the use of different, but compatible, colors, etc. Furniture placement in multi-bedded rooms can be employed to enhance privacy. It should be noted here that long-term care residents may have just as disparate tastes in furnishings as the general population. Indeed, residents have been interviewed who expressed a great liking for their very modern furnishings and even super graphics found in a New England long-term care facility.

Beds

Beds may be adjustable in height through a certain range, in two elevations only, or may be fixed in height. Height adjustments may be made manually by releasing telescoped legs, by a hand-crank, or electrically; the most expensive is the electrically operated. The springs can also be made adjustable, so that the head and/or foot of the bed can be raised (referred to as gatch springs or double gatch springs).

Beds are also available with side-rails to prevent confused residents from falling out of bed. Mattresses should always have waterproof ticking. Some mattresses are also available with a germicide impregnated in the ticking, the value of which may be subject to question.

The value of a multi-height bed lies in being able to raise it for the convenience of a nurse performing some treatment on a bedridden resident. The extra convenience of a multi-height bed is expensive and adds an institutional quality to the appearance of the beds. Also adding to the institutional appearance are side-rails and the crank for the gatch springs; however, both are, in all probability, necessary.

Chairs

The resident's chair should have a high back, be waterproof and easily cleanable. Padded arms are necessary for safety and comfort and to assist the resident in rising up or lowering himself into the seat.

Other Furnishings

A resident may be fed from an overbed table, or he may use it to read from. It should be adjustable in height and tiltable.

The resident needs a bedside cabinet in which he may store toilet articles, and this cabinet can also be used to store a bedpan, urinal and/or emesis basin.

Built-ins or wardrobes are available for clothes storage. Each resident should be provided with a lockable cabinet or drawer.

In multi-bedded rooms, cubicle curtains are required in order to make a bed private when a resident is undergoing a treatment or using a bedpan.

Each resident sleeping room should have a mirror installed in such a way as a resident can see himself, whether standing or seated, as in a wheelchair. Mirrors promote good grooming and are an aid in reality orientation.

In areas used by residents elsewhere in the facility, tables should be of sufficient height to allow use by wheelchair-bound residents and seating should have the same qualities as previously stated.

SIGNAGE AND GRAPHICS

Most long-term care facilities are fairly complex buildings. The orientation of visitors, residents and workers becomes a complicated problem requiring a creative solution. Signage, like all the other components, must reinforce the total concept of the facility and must work together to project the desired image. This means the signage should be developed in the design stage and not after the building is occupied. Signs are a simple means to lead people through unfamiliar areas. People feel more comfortable having a sense of direction.

Exterior Signs

Exterior signs are needed to identify the building, entrances and exits to parking lots and to direct the visitors around and into the facility.

Interior signs

Interior signage is generally more involved. The following is a general list of the signs found in a long-term care facility:

- Directory: The first reference point needed after entering the building. This should include specific instructions on how to get to every part of the building. The directory may include a simplified floor plan of the building.

- "Road Signs": These signs will help directing people to the proper areas or departments.

- Room Identification: All doors will have to have some identification or at least a number. Resident room identification is essential, and the room numbers should be raised and in high color contrast to help those with visual disabilities. Some signs are available which allow space to affix the resident's name, stamped in relief on an adhesive tape or by other method.

- Disaster Evacuation Chart: Regulations require that a schematic drawing of the building be posted in various locations in the facility indicating the nearest emergency exit.

The days of the handpainted signs are long gone, but still there are problems with having custom-made signs in an institutional building, since frequent changes will make them obsolete. The best solution is to select a sign system that will degenerate into handwritten messages or inconsistent, ready-made signs.

Symbols can supplement or replace verbal signs. Some are done in three dimensional relief to perform as universal communicating devices, regardless of language, literacy or even vision limitations of residents and visitors. Probably the most effective system would be to combine symbols with appropriate verbiage. Both symbols and verbiage should employ high contrast colors, simple raised letters which will facilitate reading by even the blind, if the letters can be touched. Federal regulations require that some signs be of raised letter construction such as those which identify rooms or offices. These signs must be placed on the wall to the left or right of the door at a height between 4 feet 6 inches and 5 feet 6 inches from the floor.

The use of good signage and graphics is a valuable aid to reality orientation. Most facilities have reality orientation boards to remind the residents of some basic facts. These generally are homemade signs that could undergo some improvements.

[handwritten margin note: signage must be closer to ground for wheel chair people. htw 4'6" → 5'6"]

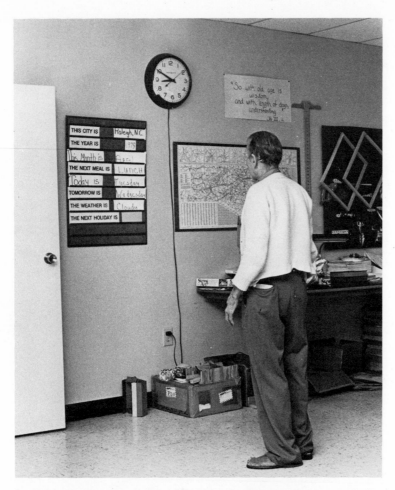

Reality Orientation Board. Note the use of the clock and the map as further aids to orientation. (*Photographer: Bobby Thompson*)

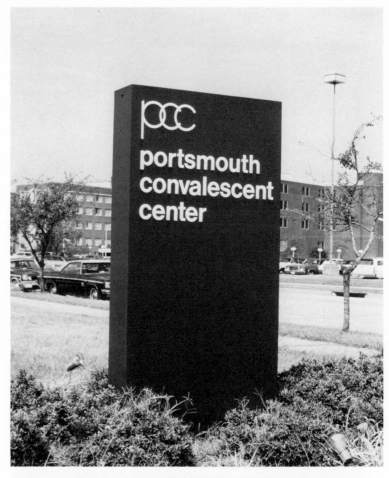

Simple, well designed exterior sign. (*Courtesy Architectural Graphics, Inc.*)

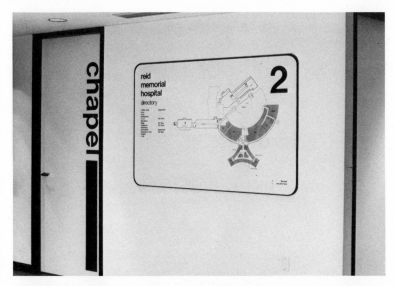

Directory including a simplified plan of the building. (*Courtesy Architectural Graphics, Inc.*)

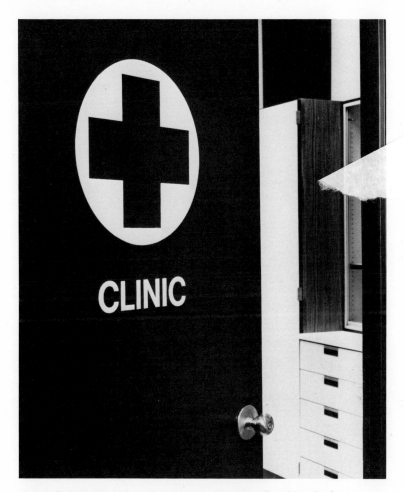

Room identification sign. (*Courtesy Architectural Graphics, Inc.*)

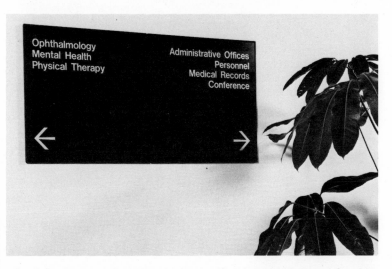

"Road Sign" giving directions to people. (*Courtesy Architectural Graphics, Inc.*)

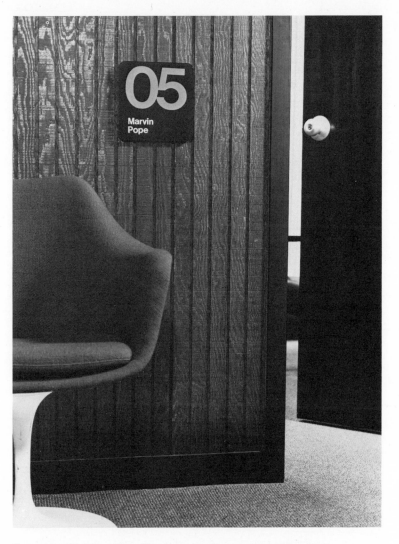

Room identification sign. (*Courtesy Architectural Graphics, Inc.*)

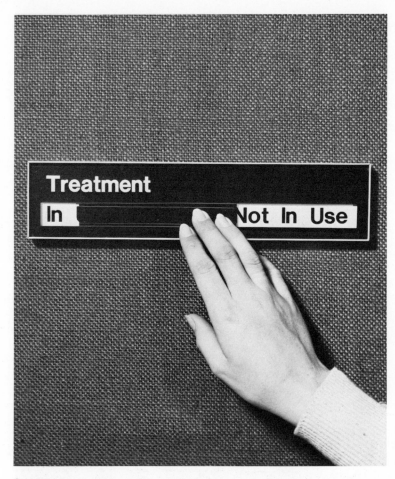

Special sign to indicate if room is in use or not. (*Courtesy Architectural Graphics, Inc.*)

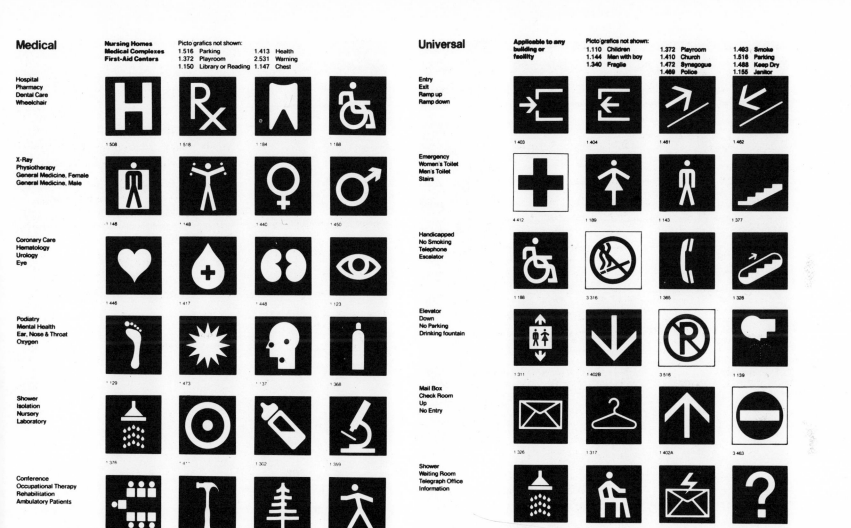

Medical

	Nursing Homes Medical Complexes First-Aid Centers	Picto grafics not shown: 1.516 Parking 1.413 Health 1.372 Playroom 2.531 Warning 1.150 Library or Reading 1.147 Chest		
Hospital Pharmacy Dental Care Wheelchair	1 508	1 518	1 184	1 188
X-Ray Physiotherapy General Medicine, Female General Medicine, Male	1 146	148	1 440	1 450
Coronary Care Hematology Urology Eye	1 446	1 417	1 448	1 123
Podiatry Mental Health Ear, Nose & Throat Oxygen	129	473	37	1 368
Shower Isolation Nursery Laboratory	1 376	4	1 302	1 359
Conference Occupational Therapy Rehabilitation Ambulatory Patients			1 480	152

Visual symbols (called picto'graphics) for medical facilities to supplement written messages. (*Courtesy Architectural Graphics, Inc.*)

Universal

	Applicable to any building or facility	Picto'grafics not shown: 1.110 Children 1.372 Playroom 1.483 Smoke 1.144 Man with boy 1.410 Church 1.516 Parking 1.340 Fragile 1.472 Synagogue 1.488 Keep Dry 1.469 Police 1.155 Janitor		
Entry Exit Ramp up Ramp down	1 403	1 404	1 461	1 462
Emergency Women's Toilet Men's Toilet Stairs	4 412	1 189	1 143	1 377
Handicapped No Smoking Telephone Escalator	1 188	3 316	1 365	1 328
Elevator Down No Parking Drinking fountain	1 311	1 402B	3 516	1 139
Mail Box Check Room Up No Entry	1 326	1 317	1 402A	3 463
Shower Waiting Room Telegraph Office Information	1 376	1 151	1 327	1 530

General purpose visual symbols (called picto'graphics) (*Courtesy Architectural Graphics, Inc.*)

29

PROFILE OF LONG-TERM CARE FACILITY RESIDENTS

Based mostly on a study conducted by the U.S. Department of Health, Education and Welfare in 1975, the following is an abbreviated profile of the long-term care facility residents.

Age:	78% 65 years or older 50% 80 years or older 11% 90 years or older
Sex Ratio:	Women outnumber men by about 3 to 1.
Education:	About 70% of the nursing home residents have an eighth grade education or less, and 10% had no schooling at all. This situation is expected to improve greatly in the future.
Family Income:	68% had less than $3,000 per year, 22% had no income at all. This indicates 90% were below poverty level.
Communication:	18% cannot communicate at all; 7% communicate nonverbally.
Orientation:	54% are disoriented (unaware of time, place and their identity).
Behavior:	41% exhibited some behavioral problems. Out of these about one-third were "wanderers," creating security and safety problems.
Bladder and Bowel Functions:	About 60% of the residents have difficulty with one or both.
Sight:	67.8% had some impairment and 2.6% were legally blind.
Hearing:	31.4% had hearing impairment; 1.5% did not hear at all.
Speech:	23.3% had some speech impairment; 8.7% did not speak at all.
Mobility:	More than half of the residents needed assistance with walking.
Dressing:	72% of the residents required the assistance of another person when dressing.
Eating:	50% of the residents required some kind of assistance in order to eat.
Bathing:	94% required either partial or complete assistance with bathing.
Toileting:	68% of the residents need assistance with toileting (getting to and from the toilet room, transferring on and off the toilet, cleansing self and arranging clothes).
Illness:	Many of the residents have more than one illness. The most common ones: Chronic Brain Syndrome Stroke Fractures Neurological Disease Diabetes Diseases of Musculoskeletal System
Length of Stay in Long-Term Care Facility:	Some residents stay as long as 10 to 15 years; the average is somewhere between 5 to 7 years.

LIGHTING

Well-designed lighting, artificial and natural, is essential in a long-term care facility. It increases the safety factor by decreasing the chances of accidents and equalizes visual opportunity for those with substandard vision. Good lighting also helps create a positive and aesthetically pleasing environment for the residents, staff and visitors. In lighting design, we must bear in mind that the elderly resident population will have reduced sensory perception. They are unable to see details in dim light, and their eye is slow to adapt to varying intensities of light.

To attain a balanced visual system concerned with comfort and efficiency, it is necessary to design both the electric lighting and the day-lighting against the same criteria. The goal in both cases is the production of a glare-free, visual environment, where brightness-balance is appropriate to the activity performed. A basic rule-of-thumb to follow concerning illumination is to provide a proper artificial lighting system, as if no other lighting source were available. The least desirable systems are those where the sources of light are of small physical dimensions and are coupled with dark ceiling areas between light sources. Direct lighting systems are improved with the use of good polarizing panels, instead of lenses or simple diffusers, or with the use of high angle, cut-off diffusers. In small rooms (resident rooms, offices, examining rooms, etc.) conventional ceiling light sources are generally satisfactory for providing adequate overall lighting, as long as task lighting is provided at desks, beds, and grooming areas. If incandescent lamps are used for general lighting, indirect light fixtures provide the most suitable quality. Illumination levels for incandescent lighting systems are usually limited, due to the heat produced and the energy consumed. Fluorescent lighting is preferred to incandescent when the lamp is exposed to the task, as in louvered-bottom direct lighting systems.

Glare and Contrast

The difference between quality and quantity of light must be stressed. A sufficient quantity (footcandles) of light is important, but other factors such as glare, color rendering properties and light distribution play a very important role in the visual environment.

Glare is excessive brightness and is of two types: direct and reflected. Direct glare, light the eye sees directly, is commonly

caused by windows and lighting fixtures. Reflected glare is brightness which the eye sees reflected from a surface. Reflected glare is set at a minimum when the area producing light is maximum, or when the contrast between the ceiling and the lighting fixture is minimum. Glare is distracting and annoying and can cause pain.

Our eye adapts when it fixes on a task. Any change in brightness-level requires a readaptation of the eye. The elderly have difficulty in eye recovery when moving from a lighted area to a dark area and vice versa. Abrupt changes in lighting levels or types should be avoided or at least mitigated with transitional lighting arrangements. We should remember that most visual tasks are seen by reflected light. Depending on the character of the task, reflected glare may or may not be a problem, but it should definitely be considered.

[handwritten margin note: direct glare caused by windows + lighting fixtures reflected by reflected off surface (may not be a prob- most light we see is reflected)]

Light Sources

The selection of light sources for a given functional area should be based on several criteria, some apparently contradictory. The most obvious is that of providing high, glare-free lighting levels, which is necessary for resident's safety, and keeping the cost of operation of lighting at a minimum. This end can be accomplished by limiting the use of incandescent lighting and making more use of the more efficient light sources, such as fluorescent, metal halide, high pressure sodium and, to a limited degree, mercury vapor. Based on color characteristics, fixture availability, lamp wattage limitatons, lamp life and function of space to be illuminated, the use of the higher efficiency lamps should be considered.

Color

[handwritten note: color of skin can change w/lighting = misdiagnosis]

Color, as produced by the light source and the surroundings, is an important consideration in some areas. For example, physicians sometimes make diagnoses based on changes in color of the resident's skin; however the color of the light can effect the skin color as perceived by the physician. In nearly all parts of the facility, the colors resulting from lighting and wall finishes should be used to alleviate the institutional appearance and to give the impression of home. Room and area atmospheres can be "softened" or "warmed-up" with the use of proper light sources. Lamps which emit light predominantly in the yellow to red range of the spectral energy distribution chart have the greatest tendency to "warm-up" rooms. The effect can be enhanced through the use of incandescent, color improved fluorescent or high pressure sodium light sources. If high pressure, sodium lamps are selected, the color scheme used by the designer must be carefully coordinated, since this light source will alter most colors, except yellow.

In areas where color quality (rendition) is important, the light source should be kept as close as possible to that of natural daylight by using color improved fluorescent, high intensity discharge or incandescent lighting. For economy of energy, high efficiency lights can be used to raise the general lighting levels, together with good color rendering lights where color quality is essential.

It is known that in most humans, the color most easily perceived is in the yellow region of the spectral distribution chart. With this in mind, the use of colors having yellow in them and light sources peaking in the yellow region, such as high pressure sodium, should enable one to see easily.

Exterior Lighting

For a facility such as this, exterior lighting is of great importance. Carefully planned, tasteful exterior lighting will avoid a depressing, institutional appearance and enhance safety. By extending the view of residents, it promotes a feeling of well-being and security.

The following are the recommended lighting levels for outdoor areas:

Parking	1 footcandle
Walks	1 footcandle
Steps	4 footcandles
Entrances	4 footcandles

AUXILIARY ELECTRICAL SYSTEMS

Several auxiliary systems must be incorporated in order to provide proper safety and security for the residents and employees. Most states now require that the majority of the following systems be included in the renovation or new construction of a long-term care facility.

Fire Alarm System

Obviously, the fire alarm system is of paramount importance in a long-term care facility. The system should incorporate basic features that include, but are not limited to, the following:

- The system must be capable of detecting fires in areas likely to have flammable contents, be primarily uninhabited or unsupervised, or occupied primarily by residents.
- The most common fire detection devices utilize photo-cell type smoke detectors. In the boiler room a "rate-of-rise" heat detector is used.
- The alarm should annunciate throughout the facility all alarm conditions, indicating the probable presence of fire. It is preferable, and in most localities required, that the local police and/or fire department be automatically notified of an alarm condition.
- The alarm annunciation should be such that facility supervisory staff and fire fighters have no problem locating the origin of the alarm condition.
- The system should automatically and constantly supervise its own status.
- Manual pull stations should be located at the exits and at the nurses station.

Nurse Call System

The primary function of the nurse call system is to enable a relatively small nursing staff to be on call to a relatively large number of residents. The system should have provisions for two-way communication between the residents' bed location and the nurses' station and, in addition, an emergency call button to be located in the residents' toilet, bath and shower rooms. In order to aid the locating of the calls, each resident's room and the head of each corridor (if several

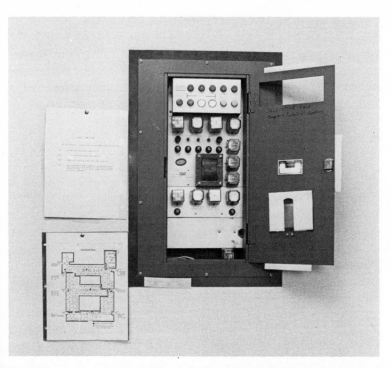

Fire alarm system central station. A light would indicate general location of the fire. Note fire evacuation plan next to station. (*Photographer: Bobby Thompson*)

Emergency Power System

The need for an emergency power system is obvious in a facility such as this. The safety, security and minimum comfort of the residents should be provided for in the event that the normal electrical system becomes inoperative due to electric utility company failure, adverse weather conditions, equipment failure, vandalism, etc. The system should be capable of going into the emergency power mode automatically and within 10 seconds. In order to insure an acceptable level of availability, the system should periodically be automatically test run under load.

The electrical loads which should be included on the emergency power system (most are required by law) are as follows:

- Lighting required for safe and orderly egress and for the nurses' station normal operation
- Complete fire alarm system
- Nurse call system
- Fire suppression system (if electrically operated)
- Elevators (at least one)
- Security systems
- Telephone and intercommunication systems
- Heating system for residents' rooms

corridors occur within a single nursing station) should have an illuminated device which indicates the origin of the call. The calls must register at the nurses' station and have a visible signal in the clean utility room, soiled utility room and the nourishment station.

Door Security System

When the layout of the facility dictates it, a door security and alarm system may be advisable. If the facility is in a high vandalism locality, and the exterior doors are not readily in sight of the nursing staff, a door alarm system may be necessary. Also, if the exterior doors are not easily supervised, or if they are large in number, a door security system may be required. This system could allow local and remote locking and unlocking of exterior doors normally accessible to residents and, if desired, annunciation of which doors are open or closed.

Telephone System

The governing body will have to decide if the equipment will be leased from the public telephone company or purchased from a private vendor. In many instances, it has been found that outright purchases of the equipment is more economical. Before a decision can be made, the following will have to be considered:

- Cost of maintenance
- Cost of moving instruments
- Insurance
- Capital investment
- Property taxes

A decision will have to be made as to whether the resident rooms will have telephone connections, and if these will go through a central switchboard. The resident rooms can have private telephones with individual, direct billing.

There are many telephone lines required in a long-term care facility, and the location of the central switchboard must be carefully considered. When the offices close for the day, one of the nurses stations can answer outside calls.

The internal communication system is generally integrated with the telephone system. Incidentally, some of the newer facilities use portable pagers to replace the usual public address system announcements. The reason is, again, to lessen the institutional atmosphere.

The telephone equipment will take a rather large wall space of approximately 8 feet by 8 feet in, or near, the mechanical room.

Television Antenna System

In most instances, a central television antenna will be required. An empty conduit system should be provided in the building construction contract with outlets in resident rooms, lounges, etc. If there is cable T.V. in the locality, the company furnishing this service should be contacted for additional technical recommendations.

CLIMATE CONTROL

General

Human beings can only exist within a narrow range of environmental limits. The generally frail condition of long-term care facility residents dictates the necessity for stringency in comfort criteria and control flexibility. This comfort criteria is not limited to temperature but must also include control of humidity in order to avoid respiratory illness, dehydration and static electricity problems, as well as good quality air sanitation to prevent the spread of odors, air pollutants and bacteria.

It is found that the elderly are more likely to complain of being too cold than too warm; usually 5°F higher temperature is needed by the elderly. Additionally, older people are affected more severely by extremes in both heat and cold. Death rate from heat stroke rises rapidly above age 60.

The load characteristics for equipment design of long-term care facilities are typified by the following:

- 24-hour per day, 7-day per week operation
- low occupancy concentration; relatively few people occupy a large building
- light or sedentary activity in resident areas
- occasional heavy occupancy, smoking in dining rooms
- large exterior exposure; long-term care facilities have a lot of outside walls because the bedrooms need windows
- shifting interior loads: The same number of people move around in the building
- large kitchen appliance loads
- high domestic water load
- the permanence of occupancy and 24-hour a day usage provides higher load factors which means larger equipment capacity requirements

Large kitchen appliance loads, high domestic water loads and the necessity, at times, for the use of systems which must sacrifice economy in energy consumption in order to provide required environmental control make these facilities an excellent candidate for energy profile studies, along with internal source heat recovery and total energy systems.

System Considerations

The design engineer is generally concerned with five functional areas:

- Resident areas
- Administrative and support facilities
- Treatment areas and special medical services
- Clean work areas, storage and supply distribution
- Soiled work areas, collection and sanitizing

System selection should be made on the basis of its ability to maintain environmental criteria. This criteria should be established based on local, state and federal requirements and the design engineers own experience. Generally, design conditions will fall within the criteria indicated for specific rooms later on in this book. It must be kept in mind that the indicated temperature, humidities and pressure relationship are recommendations only and represent an average of summer and winter temperatures that fall within the usual range of conditions. The designer should refer to the above mentioned agencies and industry standards for final determination of actual criteria utilized in system design.

System selection and air distribution should also give consideration to minimizing draft and noise. Air movement should be limited to 40 feet per minute. Generally, higher noise levels can be tolerated by residents when the noise is constant, whereas intermittent or cycling-type noises must be held to lower levels.

Odor Control By Mechanical Means

The spread of odors, air pollutants and bacteria may be limited by the use of high efficiency filters. Bacterial levels in long-term care facilities are not so critical as that experienced in hospitals. Odor control can normally be achieved by adhering to exhaust requirements within a space and by maintaining proper pressure relationships between adjacent rooms. Clean or sterile areas should be maintained at a positive or higher pressure than adjacent areas to insure against the flow of contaminated air into the space. Conversely unclean areas shall be maintained at a negative or lower pressure than surrounding areas to prevent air flow into clean areas. Other spaces are usually maintained at a pressure equal to adjacent areas. (Also see ''Odor Control'').

Available Systems

The types of systems utilized in long-term care facilities run the full gamut from constant temperature, variable volume systems to multiple unitary systems (like through-the-wall units). The potential of these systems for providing quality air cleaning and air distribution varies from excellent to poor. It is generally recognized that of all air systems with mixtures of return and outside air, high efficiency filters have the best potential for providing the required features. Air-water systems are somewhat limited in their ability to meet these requirements and multiple unitary and all water systems cannot meet these requirements at all, unless used with supplementary systems. Systems which cannot maintain desired design criteria are not recommended for long-term care facilities, although their use is common in low cost installations. No matter what type of system is utilized it must be kept in mind that it will not perform as designed over an extended length of time without proper maintenance. The use of micro-processors and even computers is becoming more common in larger facilities to provide constant monitoring of all components of the system with capabilities to reset temperatures, close or open dampers as required for efficient operation and energy conservation.

PLUMBING

The design of plumbing system for long-term care facilities differs from other multiple residential facilities in its high hot water usage due to having a commercial kitchen, laundry, sanitizing and other general purpose usages. A greater variety of water temperatures are required as well. Temperatures in areas occupied by or accessible to residents are limited to 110°F, but 180°F water must be available for sterilization in laundries, kitchen and utility areas. Because of their high use characteristics, these facilities are excellent candidates for the utilization of solar energy for domestic water heating with good pay-back potential.

Fixtures

There are special plumbing fixtures available for long-term care facilities:

Lavatory: Gooseneck faucets should be provided for all hand washing lavatories; the valves should be controlled by foot, knee or wrist to prevent contamination. The lavatory itself should be of the barrier-free type in at least half of the rooms.

Toilet Fixtures: Bedpan cleaning device is required in the private toilets; the fixture itself should be of the barrier-free type

Bathing Facilities: Hydraulic lift equipped tub is the most desirable, otherwise an elevated bathtub or a shower will be used; showers should be fitted with spray heads on flexible hoses.

Clinical Service Sink: Similar to a water closet but used for emptying liquid waste from bedpans; this is usually located in the soiled utility room.

Equipment Washer-Sanitizer: This equipment is similar to the residential dishwasher but designed for medical use.

Sterilizer: This is a large covered container in which hospital type utensils are placed under water and heated to boiling temperature.

Vacuum breakers and back flow preventers must be installed on a great number of plumbing fixtures. Consult applicable codes for requirements.

Sprinkler System

A sprinkler system is generally mandatory for all long-term care facilities. The system should be designed for light hazard occupancy and interlocked with the building fire alarm system; the main sprinkler valve must be monitored.

36

ACOUSTICS

Acoustical control in the long-term care facility is important, because certain sounds can be comforting, but excessive noise produces irritation, distraction, and fatigue in residents. Older people are unable to hear conversation clearly when there is background noise, such as from appliances, air conditioning units, or other people in active conversation. The level at which a constant background noise is acceptable is usually defined as that level which is consistent with the ability to hear normal speech easily. Some acoustical problems in buildings are caused by the following:

- Trend toward large spaces without divisions: just the opposite of the accepted concept of acoustical privacy.
- Buildings have more equipment, especially heating and air conditioning equipment.
- Lighter construction materials to save space and cost: Weight is one of the most important aspects of sound enclosure.
- Openings and joints in walls permit the harmful transmission of sound.

Noise

All sounds that are annoying are looked upon as noise. There are two categories of noise:

External noise
Internal noise

External noises are generated by the following:

Highway traffic
Construction equipment
Mechanical equipment
Aircraft

Internal noises are generated by many sources:

Mechanical and electrical equipment noises:
Pumps
Fans
Air conditioning
Heating

Light fixtures
Elevators
Escalators
Door operators

Personnel activity noises:
Resident activities
Footsteps in corridors
Speech noises
Opening and closing of doors
Public address system

Equipment noises:
Computers
Office machines
Televisions, radios, background music system
Garbage disposer
Laundry equipment
Kitchen equipment
Housekeeping equipment

Noise Control

There are many ways noise can be controlled, reduced or completely eliminated:

Controlling Noise at the Source: This is the cheapest way to control noise. This can be accomplished by purchasing quiet machines, properly maintaining equipment or by simply instructing personnel to be more careful in closing doors.

Site Planning: It is difficult to eliminate external noises, but the effect can be reduced by careful placement of the building. If possible, the structure should be set back as far as possible from noisy streets.

Architectural Design: Building elements should be divided into quiet and noisy groups, horizontally and vertically. Windows and doors should be placed to avoid direct sound paths from one to another.

Mechanical and Electrical Design: Noise and vibrations producing equipment should be placed in a basement or otherwise isolated from quiet areas. Recessed fixtures and outlet boxes in walls should always be staggered to avoid sound transmission.

Sound Absorption: If the noise source cannot be controlled, an attempt should be made to absorb the sound by using acoustical materials on the wall and ceiling surfaces and in the construction of the walls surrounding the space in question.

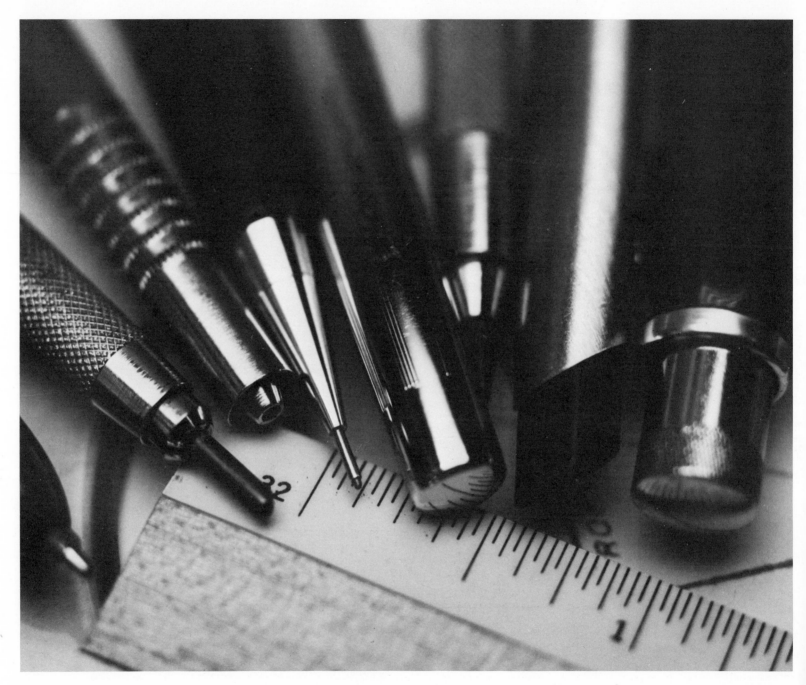

4.
Detailed Design Considerations

This section contains a great deal of information to help the designer understand the inner workings of a long-term care facility. The model selected was a 120-bed facility, this being the most popular size from the standpoint of economy of construction and management. Larger facilities should be considered as a multiple of 120 beds or a multiple of a single nursing unit, which may be anywhere from 30 to 60 beds. We have tried to list as many considerations as possible under the individual headings; however, we know people will find additional items that we have missed or sometimes completely disagree with our choices. Some of the headings require some explanations, while most of them are self-explanatory.

NUMBER OF USERS

The purpose here is to help in sizing the space, consequently the numbers listed mean the greatest expected number of *simultaneous* users.

PRIMARY USERS

Primary users are the people for whom the space is designed.

SECONDARY USERS

Secondary users may visit the room from time to time to help others, clean the room or maintain equipment, etc., but will not "use" it for the intended, primary purpose. In addition to the ones listed, there are others who may occasionally enter the room: government inspectors, outside repairmen, "contract" service employees, pest control people, etc.

SPACE CONFIGURATION

If a room size is given, it is understood to be for a 120-bed facility. Room sizes may have to be changed for a building with higher bed capacity or additional rooms could be added to compensate for the increased requirements.

INTERIOR SURFACES

For practical reasons only the most common finishes are listed and this should only serve as a guide and not as a limitation on the designer. When unfinished surfaces are listed, like gypsum wallboard or masonry, it is assumed that these will receive two coats of paint.

MOVABLE EQUIPMENT AND FURNITURE

Items listed here will be specified by the interior designer or furnished by the users of the facility.

BUILT-IN EQUIPMENT

Generally, items listed here will be a permanent part of the building and be specified by the architect. The following items are not listed in the individual sections: electrical receptacles/switches, sprinkler heads, thermostats and smoke detectors.

CLIMATE CONTROL

Local practice and code requirements must be considered; refer to "Climate Control" for more details.

LIGHTING

Requirements and recommendations for lighting design do change from time to time; for a more detailed discussion refer to the chapter on "Lighting."

ACOUSTICS

Only specific requirements are listed; for a more detailed discussion refer to the chapter on "Acoustics."

AUXILIARY SPACES

Requirements for spaces not described elsewhere in separate sections are listed here.

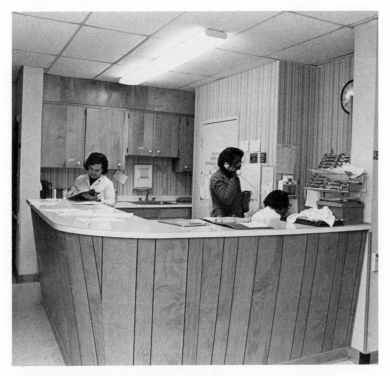

Typical nurses station in an older facility.
(Photographer: Bobby Thompson)

40

RESIDENT AREAS

Nursing Unit

Since the nurses station is the focal point of most of the activities, it is easy to understand why the residents like to stay there and "watch the traffic." In many instances, the corridor becomes the dayroom, with residents blocking the free flow of traffic when not enough space is provided.

In a well managed home most residents, unless they are too ill, are strongly urged to get out of their rooms. Then they are just as strongly encouraged to participate in the planned activities, which lessens feelings of loneliness and boredom.

The use of a desk height counter at the nurses station helps eliminate the hospital-like appearance. After all the only fixed items to be housed here are the nurse-call control panel, the fire or smoke-alarm panel and a telephone. The charts are best kept in a small adjacent room with a large, glass, vision panel for observation of the residents. The nurses, physicians and other professionals need complete privacy while doing the charting, which includes daily notes describing changes in the status of residents.

Most codes will not allow more than 60 beds per nursing unit. The recommendation is to limit the number of beds to between 40 to 50 beds. Easy view of the corridors leading to the rooms and other patient areas must be provided.

ACTIVITIES

Taking care of residents' needs
Bathing
Feeding
Transporting
Giving medication
Entertaining
Reality orientation
Keeping medical and personal records of residents
Communication
Monitoring security system
Receiving visitors
Note: If there is sufficient space provided around the nurses' station, some of the activities listed under Lounge/Dayroom and Activity Room can be accomplished here.

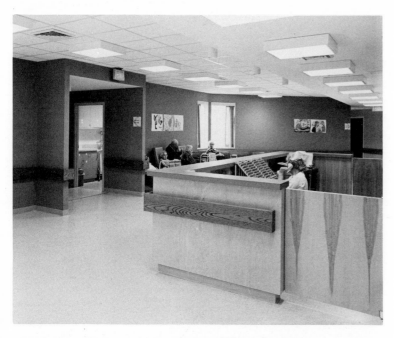

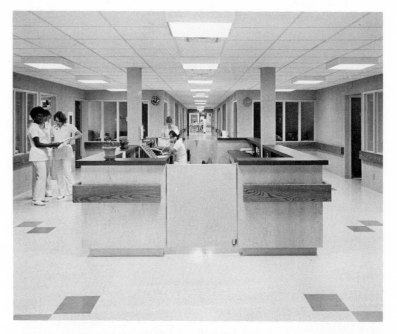

Neatly organized nurses station. Note the ample sitting area for residents to sit and watch the "traffic." (*Daughters of Sarah Nursing Home, Albany, N.Y.; Donald J. Stephens Associates, Architects*)

Specially designed nurses station for intensive care unit. (*Daughters of Sarah Nursing Home, Albany, N. Y.; Donald J. Stephens Associates, Architects*)

NUMBER OF USERS

50 to 60 people, depending on the number of beds and nursing personnel

PRIMARY USERS

Nursing personnel
Residents
Physicians
Other professionals

SECONDARY USERS

Volunteers   Housekeeping workers
Visitors   Maintenance workers
Activity workers

RELATIONSHIPS

Necessary to:	Lounge/Dayroom Resident rooms (120-foot maximum distance) Auxiliary service areas Toilets for nurses and residents
Desirable to:	Dining room Activity room Treatment rooms Outdoors
Undesirable to:	Hazardous areas Laundry Kitchen

41

ATMOSPHERE

Active
Cheerful
Stimulating

The nurses' station area should have the appearance of a reception area in an apartment building; by all means avoid the hospital look.

COLOR SCHEME

Warm color range
Primary colors for accents

SPACE CONFIGURATION

Size: 400 to 600 square feet
Ceiling height: 8 to 10 feet

INTERIOR SURFACES

Floor: Easily maintained and cleaned
                Moisture proof
                Resilient
                Durable
                Non-slip
                    Resilient tile
                    Sheet vinyl

Walls: Easily maintained and cleaned
                Washable within reach
                    Vinyl wall covering
                    Gypsum wallboard

Ceiling: Acoustical treatment recommended
                    Acoustical tile
                    Gypsum wallboard

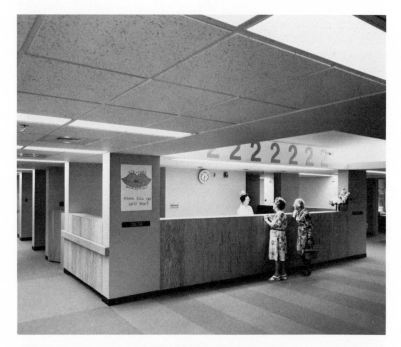

Well designed nurses station avoids the cluttered look and fits into the general decor. (*Maple Knoll Village, Springdale, Ohio; Gruzen and Partners, Architects/Planners; Photographer: Bo Parker*)

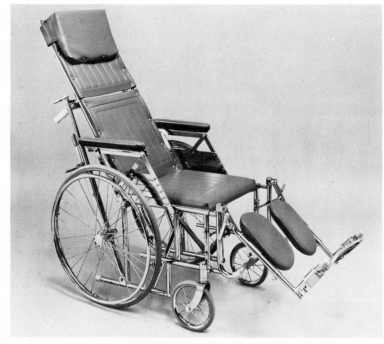

Wheelchairs come in many different forms. This is a special recliner-type with many different adjustments. (*Courtesy J. A. Preston Corporation*)

MOVABLE EQUIPMENT AND FURNITURE

Mail box	Reality orientation board
Wall clock	Wastebasket
Wall calendar	Live plants
Indoor-Outdoor thermometer	Cigarette urn (ash tray)

BUILT-IN EQUIPMENT

Desk or counter for keeping records
Drinking fountain
Bulletin board
Telephone
Public pay telephone with amplifier
Nurse-call system control panel
Security alarm control panel
Fire or smoke alarm panel
Internal communication system

CLIMATE CONTROL

Temperature:	75°F
Humidity:	30 to 50%
Outside air:	2 air changes per hour
Total air changes:	4 per hour
Pressure relationship:	Equal
	Avoid drafts

LIGHTING

Except where task lighting is needed, use soft indirect light. Natural daylight is desirable. Illumination is needed for limited office type work, such as some charting, reading of medicine labels, and other routine paperwork. Lighting levels must be adequately high for seeing tasks but not necessarily high enough to over emphasize the presence of the nurses station in its surroundings.

Quantity:	20 foot candles/general
	50 footcandles/detail
Type:	Fluorescent

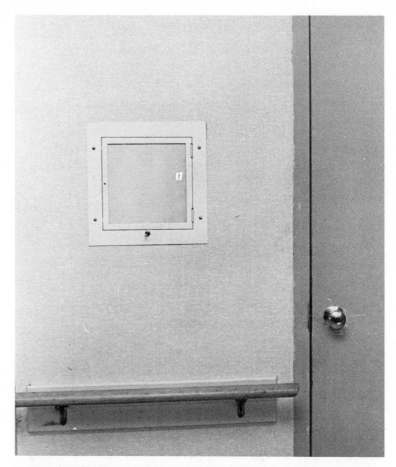

Nurse call indicator panel showing that a resident in room 17 needs assistance. (*Photographer: Bobby Thompson*)

ACOUSTICS

Reduce noise by acoustical treatment; this is one of the noisest areas in the building.

SPECIAL CONSIDERATIONS

Nursing personnel should wear some uniform but preferably not the conventional white one to promote the residential atmosphere.

Residents' public toilet: Designed to conform to "barrier-free" requirements of Nurses' toilet room.

Clean linen storage: One complete change of linens will be stored in this room. The best method is to use mobile shelving or clean linen carts. These are loaded in the laundry room and rolled to the nursing unit and stored there until needed. This room may be combined with the clean utility room.

Equipment storage room: This room is used for the storage of the following items:

Inhalators
Suction machines
Air mattresses
Walkers and similar bulky equipment
Stretchers
Wheelchairs

Janitor's closet: For storage of housekeeping supplies and equipment
Floor receptor or service sink required
All air to be exhausted directly to outdoors

Vigil room: To be located near the intensive care area for family members

Private visitation ("intercourse") room: Most facilities have no private place for the residents, if they are in a multi-bedded room. Many elderly residents would continue sexual activities if there were a place available.

Oxygen storage: A separate closet should be provided near the intensive care area, unless there is a built-in oxygen system.

The following auxiliary areas are covered in separate sections immediately following this one:

Medicine room
Clean utility room
Soiled utility room

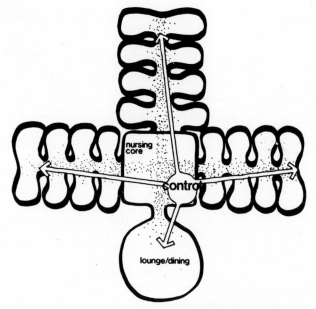

Corridor Concept

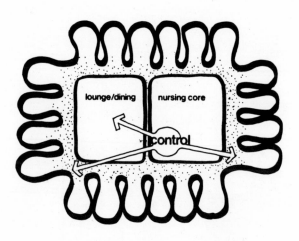

Core Concept

Nursing unit organizational concepts for the Ohio Presbyterian Homes. (*Architects: The Hoffman Partnership, Inc.*)

Medicine Room

The residents' medications are stored in this room. Because of the nature of the items stored, extra care must be taken to prevent loss. Tablets and capsules may be dispensed from capsule vials and liquid medicines from bottles, just as at home. The other method is using one of a variety of unit dose, medication systems. If the traditional method is used, cubicles must be provided for each resident for the storage of the medicines. If, however, the unit dose system is used, space in the medicine room must be provided for the storage of the unit dose medication cart. The use of the unit dose system seems to save time and reduces medication errors, making it a likely choice. This room should be adjacent to the nourishment station, because many times residents have a problem swallowing the medication; in that case, it is given to them with fruit juice or apple sauce.

ACTIVITIES

Assembling medication tray if traditional system of passing medication is employed

Inventorying of medications

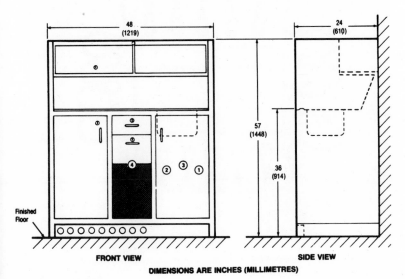

FRONT VIEW **SIDE VIEW**

DIMENSIONS ARE INCHES (MILLIMETRES)

Medicine Station

NUMBER OF USERS

1 to 2 people

PRIMARY USER

Nurses

RELATIONSHIPS

Necessary to: Nurses' station
Desirable to: Nourishment station

SPACE CONFIGURATION

Size: 50 to 60 square feet
Ceiling Height: 8 feet

INTERIOR SURFACES

Floor: Easily maintained and cleaned
                  Resilient
                  Durable
                      Resilient Tile
                      Sheet vinyl

Walls: Gypsum wallboard
                  Painted masonry

Ceiling: Acoustical tile
                  Gypsum wallboard

MOVABLE FURNITURE AND EQUIPMENT

Small refrigerator

BUILT-IN EQUIPMENT

Sink   Work counter
Lockable cabinets
One cubicle for each resident for medicine storage about 6 inches wide, 6 inches deep and 10 inches high

Ready-made compact medicine stations are available from several manufacturers.

45

CLIMATE CONTROL

Temperature:	75°F
Outside air:	2 air changes per hour
Total air changes:	4 per hour

LIGHTING

Quantity:	50 footcandles
Type:	Fluorescent

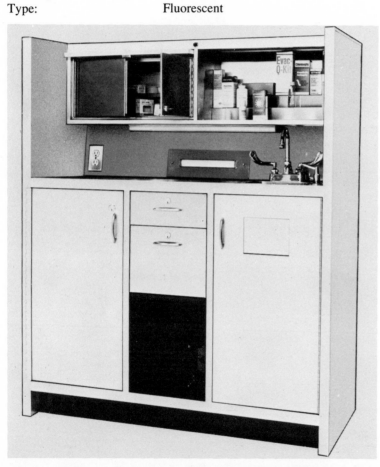

Medicine station. Compact unit includes refrigerator, narcotics compartment and warning light, sink, soap dispenser, waste compartment paper towel dispenser and lockable drawers. (*Courtesy American Sterilizer Company*)

SPECIAL CONSIDERATIONS

Room must be locked unless someone is using it.

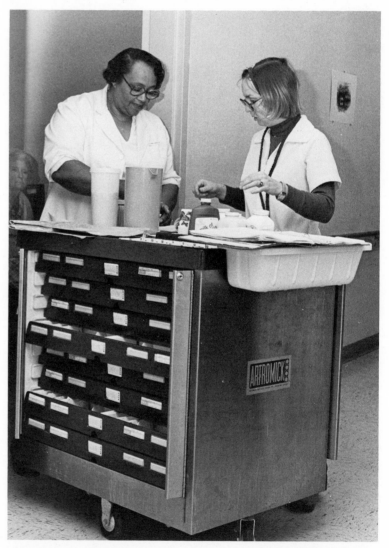

Medicine cart. Modern unit-dose medication system speeds delivery of medications to residents and minimizes errors. (*Photographer: Bobby Thompson*)

Clean Utility Room

This room is used for the storage and distribution of clean and sterile supply material.

RELATIONSHIP	
Necessary to:	Nurses' station

NUMBER OF USERS	
1 to 2 people	

SPACE CONFIGURATION	
Size:	60 to 100 square feet
Ceiling height:	8 feet

INTERIOR SURFACES	
Floor:	Resilient tile
Walls:	Gypsum wallboard Vinyl wall covering
Ceiling:	Acoustical tile

BUILT-IN EQUIPMENT	
Base and wall cabinets	Sink
Work counter	Paper towel dispenser

CLIMATE CONTROL	
Temperature:	75°F
Outside Air:	2 air changes per hour
Total air changes:	4 per hour
Pressure relationship:	Positive

LIGHTING	
Quantity:	50 footcandles
Type:	Fluorescent

Soiled Utility Room

This room is used for the disassembly of soiled equipment, disposal of liquid and solid waste, including disposable items.

NUMBER OF USERS	
1 to 2 people	

RELATIONSHIPS	
Necessary to:	Nurses' station
Desirable to:	Resident rooms

SPACE CONFIGURATION	
Size:	60 to 100 square feet
Ceiling height:	8 feet

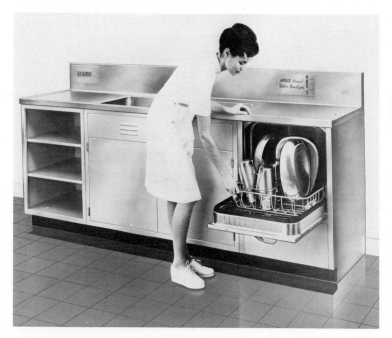

Utensil washer-sanitizer combined with counter and sink. (*Courtesy American Sterilizer Company*)

47

INTERIOR SURFACES

Floor:	Ceramic tile
Walls:	Ceramic tile
Ceiling:	Acoustical tile

MOVABLE EQUIPMENT

Waste receptacles
Soiled linen carts

BUILT-IN EQUIPMENT

Base and wall cabinets	Sanitizer
2-compartment sink	Paper towel dispenser
Work counter	

CLIMATE CONTROL

Temperature:	75°F
Outside air:	2 air changes per hour
Total air changes:	4 per hour
Pressure relationship:	Negative

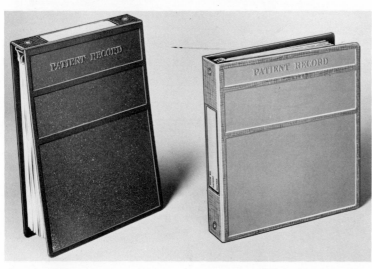

Typical patient record chart holders. (*Courtesy Carstens Health Industries, Inc.*)

LIGHTING

Quantity:	50 footcandles
Type:	Fluorescent

Charting Room

In most facilities charting is done at the nurses' station. The nurses, physicians and other professionals need privacy to do this work.

NUMBER OF USERS

2 people

RELATIONSHIP

Necessary to:	Nurses' station

SPACE CONFIGURATION

Size:	40 to 50 square feet
Ceiling height:	8 feet

INTERIOR SURFACES

Floor:	Vinyl asbestos tile
	Carpet
Walls:	Gypsum wallboard
	Vinyl wall covering
Ceiling:	Acoustical tile

MOVABLE EQUIPMENT AND FURNITURE

Desk	Charts
2 chairs	Charting supplies

BUILT-IN EQUIPMENT

Counter
Cabinets for supplies
Glass vision panel (facing nurses' station)

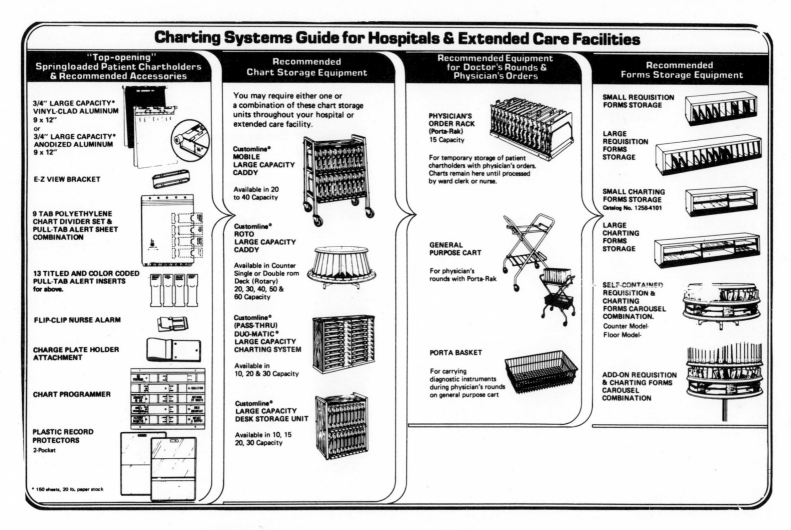

Charting Systems Guide for Hospitals & Extended Care Facilities

"Top-opening" Springloaded Patient Chartholders & Recommended Accessories

3/4" LARGE CAPACITY* VINYL-CLAD ALUMINUM 9 x 12"
or
3/4" LARGE CAPACITY* ANODIZED ALUMINUM 9 x 12"

E-Z VIEW BRACKET

9 TAB POLYETHYLENE CHART DIVIDER SET & PULL-TAB ALERT SHEET COMBINATION

13 TITLED AND COLOR CODED PULL-TAB ALERT INSERTS for above.

FLIP-CLIP NURSE ALARM

CHARGE PLATE HOLDER ATTACHMENT

CHART PROGRAMMER

PLASTIC RECORD PROTECTORS 2-Pocket

* 150 sheets, 20 lb. paper stock

Recommended Chart Storage Equipment

You may require either one or a combination of these chart storage units throughout your hospital or extended care facility.

Customline® MOBILE LARGE CAPACITY CADDY

Available in 20 to 40 Capacity

Customline® ROTO LARGE CAPACITY CADDY

Available in Counter Single or Double rom Deck (Rotary) 20, 30, 40, 50 & 60 Capacity

Customline® (PASS-THRU) DUO-MATIC® LARGE CAPACITY CHARTING SYSTEM

Available in 10, 20 & 30 Capacity

Customline® LARGE CAPACITY DESK STORAGE UNIT

Available in 10, 15 20, 30 Capacity

Recommended Equipment for Doctor's Rounds & Physician's Orders

PHYSICIAN'S ORDER RACK (Porta-Rak) 15 Capacity

For temporary storage of patient chartholders with physician's orders. Charts remain here until processed by ward clerk or nurse.

GENERAL PURPOSE CART

For physician's rounds with Porta-Rak

PORTA BASKET

For carrying diagnostic instruments during physician's rounds on general purpose cart

Recommended Forms Storage Equipment

SMALL REQUISITION FORMS STORAGE

LARGE REQUISITION FORMS STORAGE

SMALL CHARTING FORMS STORAGE Catalog No. 1258-4101

LARGE CHARTING FORMS STORAGE

SELF-CONTAINED REQUISITION & CHARTING FORMS CAROUSEL COMBINATION. Counter Model- Floor Model-

ADD-ON REQUISITION & CHARTING FORMS CAROUSEL COMBINATION

Top opening chart holders and accessories. (*Courtesy Carstens Health Industries, Inc.*)

Temperature:	75°F
Outside air:	2 air changes per hour
Total air changes:	4 per hour
Pressure relationship:	Equal

LIGHTING

Quantity:	50 footcandles
Type:	Fluorescent

SPECIAL CONSIDERATIONS

- Chart holders come in a variety of forms and they can be stored on various stands:

  Floor mounted
  Desk mounted
  Stationary
  Mobile
  Rotating

- The type of chart storage will be determined according to available space, layout, traffic flow and the particular needs of the nursing unit. Most chart storage units are available in capacities of 10 to 40 chart holders. The usual chart holder will be about 3/4-inch thick, having a 150-sheet capacity.

Nourishment Station

The purpose of this area is to serve snacks and drinks between meals. Most of the time this room is equipped like a small, residential kitchen. Ready-made nourishment center units are available from several manufacturers. These units are very sophisticated and take relatively small space but are more expensive.

NUMBER OF USERS

1 to 2 people

PRIMARY USERS

Nursing personnel

RELATIONSHIPS

Necessary to:	Nurses' station
Desirable to:	Medicine room

SPACE CONFIGURATION

Size:	60 to 80 square feet
Ceiling height:	8 feet

INTERIOR SURFACES

Floor:	Resilient tile
	Sheet vinyl
Walls:	Gypsum wallboard
	Vinyl wall covering
Ceiling:	Acoustical tile

MOVABLE EQUIPMENT AND FURNITURE

Refrigerator
Coffee maker
Blender
Waste basket

BUILT-IN EQUIPMENT

Base cabinets
Wall cabinets
Work counter
Hot plate
Sink
Microwave oven
Ice maker/dispenser
Paper towel dispenser

CLIMATE CONTROL

Temperature: 75°F
Outside air: 2 air changes per hour
Total air changes: 4 per hour
Pressure relationship: Equal
Provide exhaust fan if hot plate is used

LIGHTING

Quantity: 50 footcandles
Type: Fluorescent

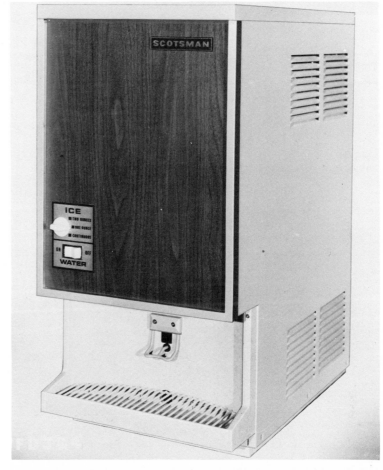

Compact countertop ice maker. One that might be used at a nourishment station with a more conventional kitchen-type arrangement. (*Courtesy Scotsman Ice Systems*)

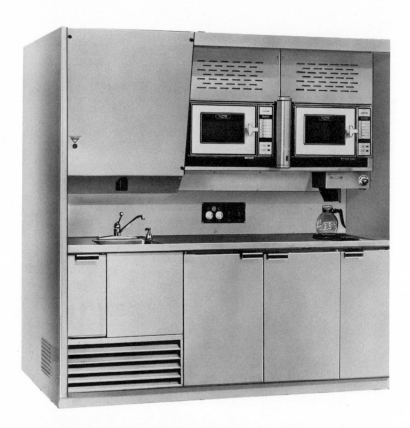

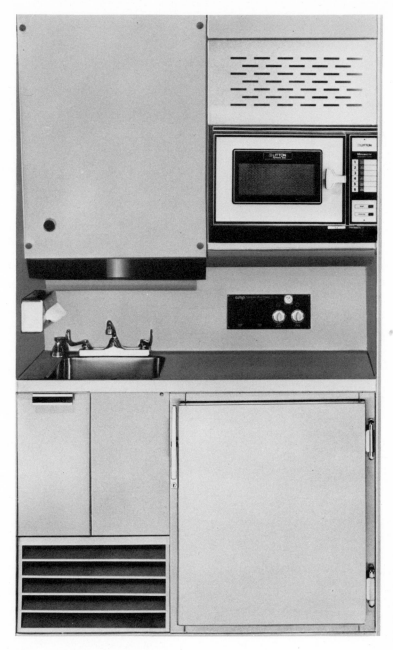

Nourishment centers. The largest of these units can include the following: paper towel dispenser, ice maker, cup dispenser, coffee maker, light, receptacles, waste container, refrigerator, freezer, hot plates, sink, microwave oven, instant hot water. These units are available in different sizes and with various equipment. (*Courtesy Continental Metal Products Co., Inc.*)

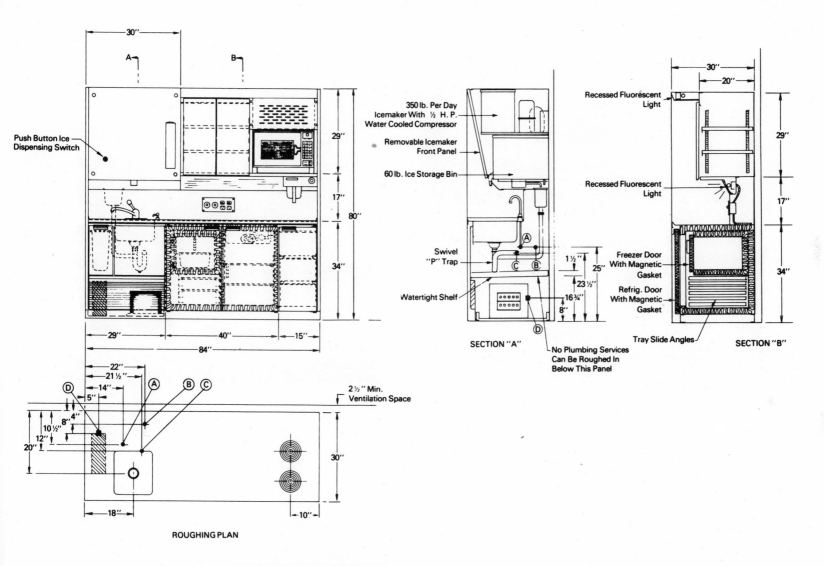

Push Button Ice Dispensing Switch

30″

A   B

29″

17″

80″

34″

29″   40″   15″

84″

22″

21½″

14″

5″

D   A   B   C

8″ 4″

10½″

12″

20″

18″

10″

30″

2½″ Min. Ventilation Space

ROUGHING PLAN

350 lb. Per Day Icemaker With ½ H. P. Water Cooled Compressor

Removable Icemaker Front Panel

60 lb. Ice Storage Bin

Swivel "P" Trap

Watertight Shelf

1½″

25″

23½″

16¾″

8″

A

C   B

D

No Plumbing Services Can Be Roughed In Below This Panel

SECTION "A"

Recessed Fluorescent Light

Recessed Fluorescent Light

Freezer Door With Magnetic Gasket

Refrig. Door With Magnetic Gasket

Tray Slide Angles

30″

20″

29″

17″

34″

SECTION "B"

Nourishment center. Detailed drawings. (*Courtesy Continental Metal Products Co., Inc.*)

Resident Rooms

Most state regulations will permit up to four residents in a sleeping room. It soon becomes obvious to the developer that the more residents are in a room, the lower the cost of construction per bed. The federal government urges "cost containment;" that is to say, the government urges developers to provide care at the lowest possible cost. The question arises, however, is this what the resident wants? If he has had any good fortune at all during his lifetime, he has been able to sleep alone or with his spouse. Communal sleeping is seldom an option for most of us, except perhaps for a tour of duty in the armed forces, where it is likely not an option but a requirement. What choice then would a resident make about his sleeping accommodations? While isolated studies have been done, little is available in print. However, sociologists suggest that the best sleeping situation is for private or semi-private accommodations.

It becomes a question of providing quality-care versus "cheap" care. The fact is that the developer is really being asked a larger question which is philosophical in nature. Will he provide an institution for the dying or a home for the living? The situation is not quite that black and white, and some compromises are possible.

While it may sound uncaring, the developer may wish to examine that segment of the population he hopes to serve. Sadly, he will find an element in our population, that would consider itself fortunate indeed to share sleeping quarters with three other persons. However, if the developer is forward looking, he will also see that this element represents a dwindling group: After all our population is becoming better educated and enjoys a steadily improving standard of living.

By providing a roommate for some residents, the developer is providing an additional safety factor; the assumption is, of course, that should one resident be unable to summon help the other might.

The Problems with Two-Bedded Rooms. The 2-bedded room does create some problems: Who gets to sleep nearest the window, door, heat or toilet? Imaginative room arrangement can provide some solutions to these problems. There are other problems: Residents frequently complain that their roommate keeps the room too hot, too cool or the television/radio too loud. Residents need an identifiable territory, which is not easy to supply; again, a little imagination can help. Residents should for instance be encouraged to personalize their rooms by doing things such as bringing in a favorite chair, a writing desk, a television, a chest of drawers, curtains or bedspreads from home or

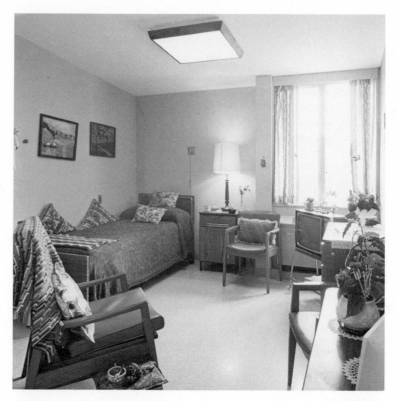

Resident room (single) allowing a great deal of individualization. (*Daughters of Sarah Nursing Home, Albany, N.Y.; Donald J. Stephens Associates, Architects*)

being allowed to hang pictures on the walls, thus creating a "territory."

The Case for Single-Bedded Rooms. Based on conversations with administrators, there is a strong preference for single rooms. Among other advantages it helps prevent conflicts between residents. Very often even married couples are best separated because of the differences in their physical and emotional conditions. Some rooms may be provided with connecting doors for the use of married couples. Incidentally, there are very few couples in institutions; according to statistics, less than 10% of the residents are married.

At least one nursing unit should include intensive care-type, single bedded rooms (2 to 3% of the total beds) with private toilets.

ACTIVITIES

Sleeping
Resting
Eating
Receiving visitors
Medical examinations
Watching television
Listening to the radio

Reading
Writing
Playing games
Pursuing hobbies or crafts
Small group socialization
Sex
Physical rehabilitation

NUMBER OF USERS

1 to 4 in single-bedded rooms
1 to 3 per bed in multi-bedded rooms

PRIMARY USERS

Residents

SECONDARY USERS

Nursing personnel
Physicians
Laboratory workers
Activity workers
Social workers
Visitors
Physical therapist

Housekeeping workers
Maintenance workers

RELATIONSHIPS

Necessary to:

Nurses' station (within 120 feet)
Toilet
Bathroom
Corridor

Desirable to:

Dining room
Lounge/Dayroom
Outdoor recreation area
Activity area
Treatment areas

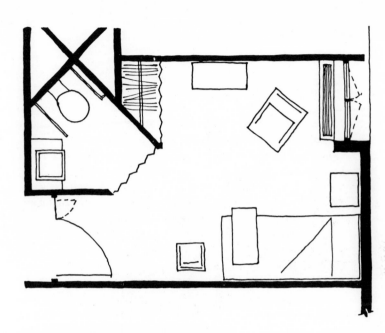

Typical resident room. (Daughters of Sarah Nursing Home, Albany, N.Y.; Donald J. Stephens Associates, Architects)

Undesirable to:

Laundry
Kitchen
Hazardous areas

ATMOSPHERE

Cheerful   Residential
Use of personal items including a piece of furniture should be encouraged.

COLOR SCHEME

Warm color range
Primary colors for accents

SPACE CONFIGURATION

Adequate room is needed for making up the bed and for residents to get around in wheelchairs. Ample space is needed (3-foot minimum)

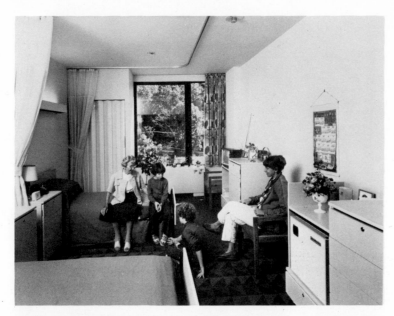

Family members visit a resident in a typical double room. (Palisade Nursing Home, Riverdale, N.Y.; Gruzen & Partners, Architects/Planners; Photographer: Nathaniel Lieberman)

around furniture. Rooms should be designed to allow a variety of furniture arrangements.

Size: (excluding closets, vestibules, wardrobes and toilet rooms):

1 bed	120 square feet
2 beds	160 to 200 square feet
3 beds	240 to 300 square feet
4 beds	320 to 400 square feet
Ceiling height:	8 feet

INTERIOR SURFACES

Floor:
Easily maintained and cleaned
Moisture proof
Resilient
Non-slip
Durable
  Vinyl asbestos tile
  Sheet vinyl

Note: Carpet is not recommended because of incontinent residents.

Walls:
Easily maintained and cleaned
Gypsum wallboard
Vinyl wall covering

Ceiling:
Gypsum wallboard
Acoustical tile

MOVABLE EQUIPMENT AND FURNITURE

Bed (fixed height, manual high-low or electric)
Photographs
Artwork
Chair (high back and arms preferred)
Over bed table
Calendar
Clock
Wastebasket
Plants
Bedside cabinet
Dresser-desk combination, some drawers to be lockable (maintenance department to have a duplicate key and the administrator to have a master key)
Movable wardrobe (may be built-in)
Cubicle curtains in multi-bedded rooms
Shades or drapes
Full length mirror

Note: Area rugs must not be permitted because of the tripping hazard.

BUILT-IN EQUIPMENT

Clothes closet
Cubicle curtain track in multi-bedded rooms
Nurse-call signaling device at the bed
Tack board (or other similar device, where residents can display photographs and other personal items without ruining the wall surface)
Telephone
Television antenna outlet
Reading light; may be portable lamp on bedside cabinet

CLIMATE CONTROL

Temperature:	75°-80°F.
Humidity:	30 to 50%
Outside air:	2 air changes per hour
Total air changes:	2 per hour
Pressure relationship:	Equal

LIGHTING

Quantity:	20 footcandles/general
	50 footcandles/detail
Type:	Incandescent

Night light required by most codes

ACOUSTICS

Acoustical treatment is recommended in areas where residents tend to be noisy. A designated area should be specially treated for "screamers." STC rating of 40 to 45 dB is recommended between adjacent rooms and 50 dB between rooms and corridor.

SPECIAL CONSIDERATIONS

- Name tags and room numbers (changeable type with raised letters for touching)
- Entrance door could be treated like the entrance to a house with exterior light fixture, door bell, mail box, etc. See "Corridors."
- Door to corridors must be 44 to 46 inches wide, solid core and without lock.
- Beds should be placed so that those bedridden residents are able to watch the activity in the corridor.
- Each room must have a window, size to equal one-eighth of the floor area, at least half of the window to be openable, window sill: 30 inches maximum recommended.

AUXILIARY SPACES

Isolation room: This room is required to control infectious diseases. Room must be single-bedded with a private toilet but other-

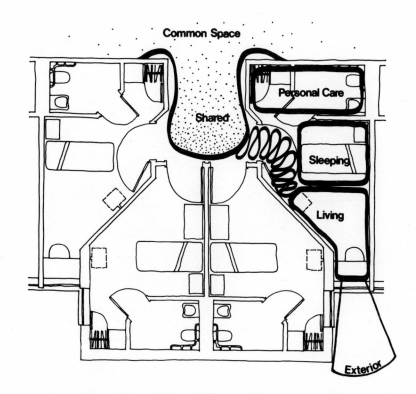

Private room organizational diagram. (*Ohio Presbyterian Homes, Willoughby, Ohio; Hoffman-Gillum, Architects/Engineers*)

wise the same as other resident rooms. All air to be either self-contained or exhausted to the exterior to prevent spreading of disease.

Intensive care room: When a resident becomes seriously ill, but does not require hospitalization, he will be transferred to this room. It must be single-bedded with a private toilet and will be identical to the other resident rooms except oxygen and suction must be provided (built-in or portable).

These rooms should be near an exit with vehicular access and close to a nurses' station. Some large facilities have a separate intensive care section with a special nurses' station.

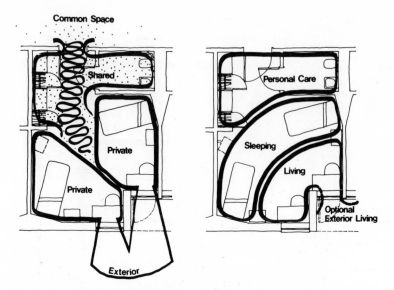

Common Space

Shared

Private

Private

Exterior

Personal Care

Sleeping

Living

Optional
Exterior Living

Semi-private room organizational diagrams. (*Ohio Presbyterian Homes, Willoughby, Ohio; Hoffman-Gillum, Architects/Engineers*)

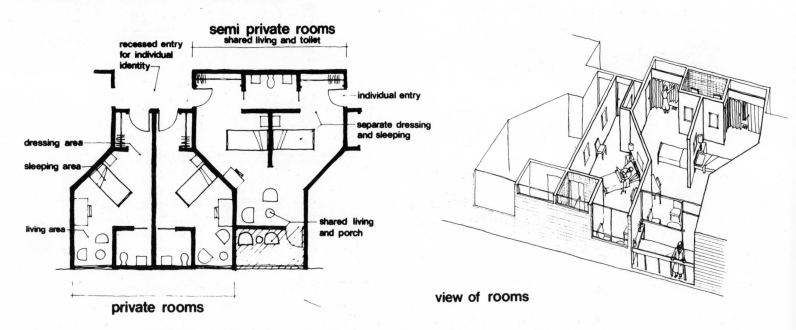

recessed entry
for individual
identity

semi private rooms
shared living and toilet

individual entry

separate dressing
and sleeping

dressing area

sleeping area

living area

shared living
and porch

private rooms

view of rooms

Resident room design study for Ohio Presbyterian Homes. (*Architect: The Hoffman Partnership, Inc.*)

58

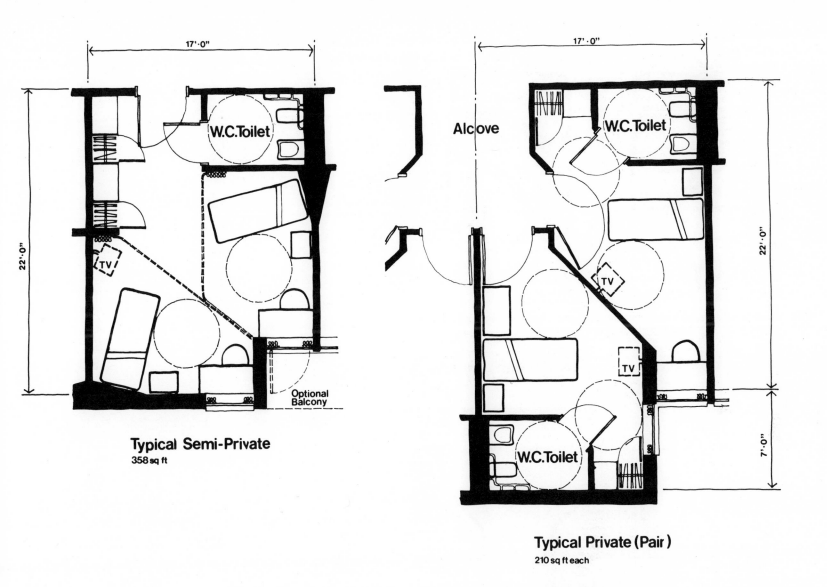

Typical Semi-Private
358 sq ft

Typical Private (Pair)
210 sq ft each

0 2 4

Private and semi-private room layouts for Ohio Presbyterian Homes. (*Architect: The Hoffman Partnership, Inc.*)

59

Resident Toilets

Toilets generally include water closet and lavatory. Most codes will allow the lavatory to be in the resident's room, but it detracts from any effort to create a residential atmosphere.

ACTIVITIES

Dressing
Personal Hygiene
Grooming
Toilet Training

NUMBER OF USERS

It is preferable to have private toilets, but most codes will allow up to four people or two bedrooms to use one toilet.

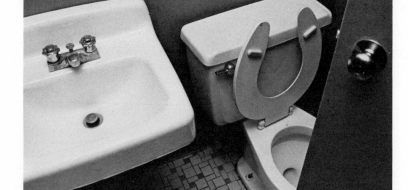

This toilet was intended for use by residents but the door cannot be fully opened, making it inaccessible to wheelchair users. (Photographer: Bobby Thompson)

PRIMARY USERS

Residents

SECONDARY USERS

Nurses
Physicians
Housekeeping workers
Maintenance workers

RELATIONSHIPS

Necessary to:

Resident rooms
Toilets must be accessible directly from the bedrooms.

ATMOSPHERE

Residential

COLOR SCHEME

Bright
Warm Colors

SPACE CONFIGURATION

Area:

5 feet by 7 feet to accommodate wheelchair-bound residents. Most codes will allow a 3- by- 6-foot room containing a water closet only; however, this does not allow enough room for a wheelchair-bound resident to turn around. Consequently, this solution is not recommended.

Ceiling Height:

8 feet

INTERIOR SURFACES

Floor: Easily maintained and cleaned
          Non-slip
              Ceramic tile
              Resilient tile

Walls: Moistureproof
          Rounded corners for safety
              Ceramic tile at least 4 feet high
              Vinyl wallcovering

Ceilings: Gypsum wallboard
          Acoustical tile

MOVABLE EQUIPMENT AND FURNITURE

Wastebasket

BUILT-IN EQUIPMENT

Water closet
Lavatory (hot water temperature: maximum 110°F)
Towel bar
Grab bars (needed on both sides for wheelchair-bound residents)
Toilet paper holder
Paper towel dispenser (used by staff and physicians)
Mirror (tilting type for wheelchair-bound residents)
Stainless steel shelf for personal articles; one for each resident using the toilet
Nurse call signaling device
All built-in equipment to conform to "barrier-free" design requirements

CLIMATE CONTROL

Temperature:	75° to 80°F
Humidity:	30 to 50%
Outside air:	Optional
Total air changes:	10 per hour
Pressure relationship:	Negative; all air is to be exhausted to outdoors

LIGHTING

Quantity:	30 footcandles/general
	50 footcandles/detail
Type:	Incandescent lighting preferred

ACOUSTICS

Some sound attenuation recommended

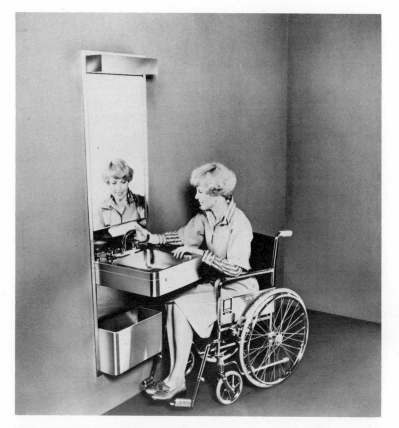

Compact washing center accessible to everyone, including handicapped persons. The unit contains light fixture, storage cabinet, mirror, towel dispenser, waste receptacle. (*Courtesy Bradley Corporation*)

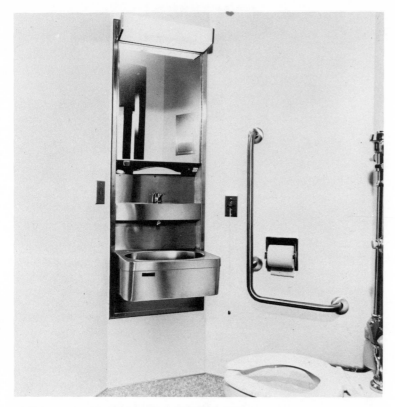

Similar to fig. on page 61 but also shows location of grab bar, toilet paper dispenser and nurse call signaling device. (*Courtesy Bradley Corporation*)

SPECIAL CONSIDERATIONS

- Door to toilet must be 3 feet wide, outswinging type, equipped with hardware to permit access in case of emergency.
- Faucets on lavatories should be lever type and have color coding (red and blue) to distinguish hot and cold water.
- All toilets in the long-term care facility used by residents should be similar to this toilet.
- Generally, not more than one-half of the residents will be in wheelchairs. This means the other one-half will not need all the "barrier-free" hardware; consequently, those toilets could be less institutional looking. Portable grab bars can be easily attached to toilets, if the need arises later on.

Residents' Lounge/Dayroom

An isolated dayroom is generally a wasted space, because the residents will not use it. The best solution is placing this room next to the nurses' station or actually combining the two functions. The residents like to see activity, and the nurses' station is busy day and night.

Lounge space is either passively or actively used by residents in nursing homes, depending on their self-help capabilities. Those able to utilize it will go to the lounge space, provided that:

- It is not removed from major traffic arteries and the nurses' station.
- Programmed activities are directed for lounge space.
- The furnishings are comfortable and, at the same time, are easily negotiated—sitting or arising.
- The furnishings are not so plentiful as to preclude wheeling one's wheelchair into the space.
- There is a toilet nearby.

Popular passive entertainment for residents is watching television. However, it seems most people end up going to sleep. One explanation for this is that the generation living in long-term care facilities today is not used to watching a great deal of television. A problem with conventional T.V. is that some residents cannot see nor hear well. Explore the use of projection-type television with individual earphones designed specifically to suit each person. These earphones could be plugged into some device like a drive-in movie stand or an overhead device similar to the ones used in a language lab.

ACTIVITIES

Sitting	Writing
Socializing	Playing games
Watching television	Eating
Reading	Receiving visitors

NUMBER OF USERS

30 to 60 residents, depending on the number of beds per nurses' station

PRIMARY USERS

Residents

SECONDARY USERS

Nursing personnel
Activity workers
Dietary workers
Visitors
Volunteers
Housekeeping workers
Maintenance workers

RELATIONSHIPS

Necessary to:
    Nurses' station
    Residents' rooms
    Toilet

Desirable to:
    Dining room
    Outdoors
    Porch

Undesirable to:
    Hazardous areas
    Administrative areas
    Lobby

ATMOSPHERE

Cheerful
Stimulating

COLOR SCHEME

Warm color range
Primary colors for accents

SPACE CONFIGURATION

Size: 15 square feet per user
Ceiling height: 8 to 10 feet

INTERIOR SURFACES

Floor:
    Easily maintained and cleaned
    Moisture proof
    Resilient
    Durable
    Non-slip
        Resilient tile
        Sheet vinyl
        Carpet (not recommended)

Walls:
    Easily maintained and cleaned
    Washable within reach
        Vinyl wallcovering
        Gypsum wallboard
        Wall carpet

Ceiling:
    Acoustical tile
    Gypsum wallboard

MOVABLE EQUIPMENT AND FURNITURE

Chairs
Tables   Calendar
Television   Wastebasket
Artwork   Reality orientation board
Clock   Cigarette urn (ashtray)

BUILT-IN EQUIPMENT

Fireplace
Nurse-call signaling device
Television antenna outlet

CLIMATE CONTROL

Temperature: 75°-80°F
Humidity: 30 to 50%
Outside air: 2 to 4 air changes per hour
Total air changes: 6 per hour
Pressure relationship: Equal

LIGHTING

Natural light through windows or skylights recommended.
Quantity: 30 footcandles
Type: Fluorescent or incandescent

ACOUSTICS

Treatment recommended to control background noise.

SPECIAL CONSIDERATIONS

The following is a list of items that could be located in the lounge to stimulate the residents:

Birdcage
Fish tank
Lava lamp
Mobile
Plants

AUXILIARY SPACES

Screened or open porch. Residents enjoy sitting outside, particularly, if they can watch the street, children's playground, sunset, etc.

Corridors

The corridors are the communication arteries of the facility. They could be developed as "streets" with individual rooms having street addresses. "Shops," such as beauty shop, barber shop, general store, and other rooms, such as the chapel, doctor's office, and activity rooms, which line the corridors, can be arranged to create a "downtown" atmosphere. This treatment will pay rich dividends in improved resident behavior and go a long way toward creating a facility for the "living."

Long corridors can be made more interesting by interrupting them with alcoves to provide resting and socializing places for residents. In poorly designed facilities, the corridors become "dayrooms," causing congestion and resident discontent.

Corridors can convey location and orientation in a facility by having signage, graphics, and color that differentiate one corridor from the next in terms of location or, more specifically, in purpose or function. Corridors can be transformed into art galleries by hanging pictures which are maintained constantly or rotated with different exhibits on a weekly, monthly or seasonal basis. Resident pictures located near room of occupancy may enhance orientation and remembrance of room number for some of the more confused population.

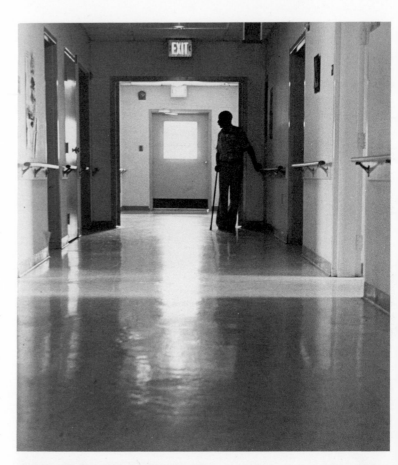

Highly reflective floors and pale colors on walls tend to be disorienting. There is a lack of definition between floor and wall. An older person with diminished sight perception will have problem seeing where one starts and the other stops. The reflection from the window may temporarily blind some people. (*Photographer: Bobby Thompson*)

ACTIVITIES

Walking
"Watching the traffic"
Chance meetings

NUMBER OF USERS

Everyone

PRIMARY USERS

Residents
Staff members

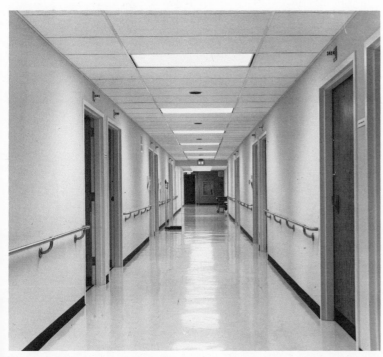

Somewhat better corridor treatment, still the lights in the middle of the ceiling cause disturbing reflections. Walls could use some decorative treatment. Handrail manufactured by Bradley Corporation. (*Courtesy Bradley Corporation*)

SECONDARY USERS

Visitors
Volunteers

RELATIONSHIPS

Necessary to: Nurses station for observation (for resident corridors only)

ATMOSPHERE

Pleasant
Avoid institutional feelings

COLOR SCHEME

Bright colors, and multi-colored graphic symbols on the wall and in the floor covering to help orient residents and staff. Avoid the use of the same color for ceilings, floors and walls. Contrasting colors on the surfaces help prevent disorientation.

SPACE CONFIGURATION

Width: 8 feet minimum in areas used by residents
5 feet minimum all other areas
Recessed doors provide more interesting space configuration

Height: 8 feet minimum

INTERIOR SURFACES

Floor: Easily maintained and cleaned
Moisture proof
Resilient
Non-slip
Durable
Sheet vinyl
Vinyl asbestos tile
Carpet (not recommended)

Walls:	Easily maintained and cleaned
	Washable within reach
	Protection from wheelchairs required
	Wall carpeting
	Vinyl wallcovering
	Gypsum wallboard
Ceiling:	Acoustical treatment recommended
	Acoustical tile
	Gypsum wallboard

MOVABLE EQUIPMENT AND FURNITURE

Artwork
Chairs (in sitting alcoves)
Directional signs
Room signs and numbers
Hanging plants
Reality orientation boards

BUILT-IN EQUIPMENT

Handrails (ends to return to walls)
Picture molding or other device to facilitate changing exhibits
Protection for walls to prevent damaging by wheelchairs
Corner guards
Internal communication system
Directional signs

CLIMATE CONTROL

Temperature:	75°F
Humidity:	30 to 50%
Outside air:	2 air changes per hour
Total air changes:	4 per hour
Pressure relationship:	Equal

LIGHTING

Do not use uniform lighting in the center of the ceilings. Indirect lighting is much better and will avoid reflections on the floor. Glare will temporarily blind people, as will windows at the end of corridors. Skylights may be used if the light is diffused. Lighting does not have to be uniform, but strong contrasts should be avoided. The lighting levels of corridors should be consistent with that of the rooms served, so that there is no objectionable light level difference in passing from one area to another. This also means that provisions must be made for reducing the levels at nighttime. From a safety standpoint, it may be desirable to control the lights with key-operated wall switches in order to minimize the possibility of a resident getting caught in a suddenly darkened corridor.

Quantity:	20 footcandles
	Night lights required by most codes to produce 3 footcandles
Type:	Fluorescent or incandescent

ACOUSTICS

There is a great deal of traffic through corridors. Treatment of walls and ceilings is recommended to avoid disturbance to residents and staff.

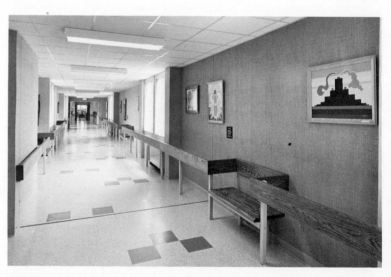

Custom-made railing is combined with benches for resting. The floor has colored tiles indicating the color code of the nursing unit ahead. Paintings on the walls and natural light create a pleasant space. (*Daughters of Sarah Nursing Home, Albany, N.Y.; Donald J. Stephens Associates, Architects*)

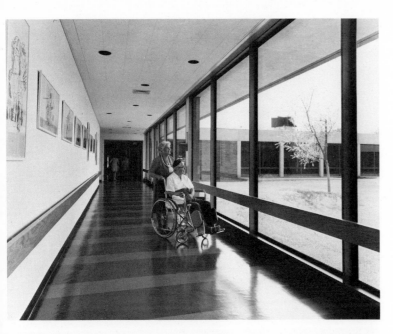

Natural light makes this corridor very cheerful. Note that the cross stripes on the floor and the random light distribution in the ceiling tend to minimize the visual length of the corridor. Pictures on the wall lend some interest to the walls; however, they seem to be placed too high, particularly for a person in a wheelchair. **(Menorah Park Jewish Home for the Aged, Beachwood, Ohio; Gruzen and Partners, Architects/Planners)**

SPECIAL CONSIDERATIONS

- Entrances can be customized to emphasize individuality by changing surface materials or by graphic methods.
- Color coding of different areas is quite helpful in orienting residents and staff, but this must be explained to the people through reality orientation and in-service training. Otherwise, they may not even be aware of the intention of the designer.

RESIDENT BATHS

In most facilities, bathing is done in large bathrooms. Even though some residents will express a preference for a private bath, it is not usually permitted, since bathing without assistance invites accidents. The solution is to provide a well equipped central bath in each nursing unit. One bath will do for both sexes, inasmuch as baths are scheduled and the residents always have an attendant present. If separate baths for men and women are desired, the designer must remember that generally there are three times as many female as male residents, which means that the facilities for men will be smaller and have fewer fixtures.

Most codes require a tub or shower for each 10 to 15 residents; this must be researched carefully, since local plumbing and state health codes may conflict and will surely vary from state to state. It should be noted, however, that showers are not very popular with residents or workers. There are a number of special tubs, even with hydraulic lifts, now available for use in long-term care facilities. Most are safer and faster than conventional tubs. They are expensive and, although faster, it is doubtful that one such tub will be allowed by state authorities to substitute for a larger number of conventional tubs (or showers). This restrictive rule might be partially overcome by using showers (which will be used only occasionally), instead of conventional tubs and use of the special tub routinely. Generally, residents are bathed once or twice a week, except incontinent residents, who are bathed as needed.

ACTIVITIES

Personal hygiene
Grooming
Dressing
Toilet training
Bathing

NUMBER OF USERS

2 people per plumbing fixture

PRIMARY USERS

Residents
Nursing personnel

SECONDARY USERS

Housekeeping workers
Maintenance workers

67

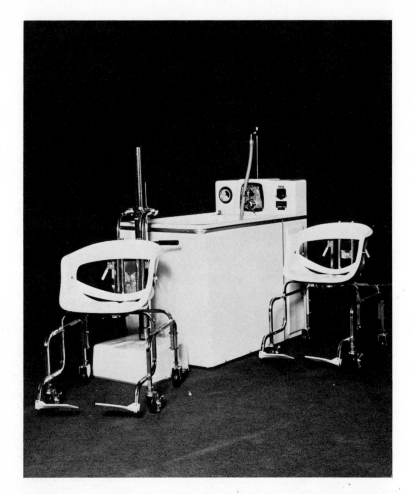

Hydraulic lift equipped bathtub. (*Courtesy of Century Manufacturing Company*)

Cheerful
Lively

COLOR SCHEME

Bright colors

SPACE CONFIGURATION

Sized for required equipment; provide ample space for movement of wheelchairs and working room for nursing personnel.

INTERIOR SURFACES

Floor:	Moisture proof
	Easily maintained and cleaned
	Non-slip
	Durable
	Ceramic tile
	Quarry tile
	Terrazzo
	Sheet vinyl and vinyl asbestos are not recommended
Walls:	Easily maintained and cleaned
	Rounded corners for safety
	Ceramic tile at least 6 feet high, recommended full height
Ceiling:	Smooth plaster
	Gypsum wallboard
	Water-resistant acoustical tile

MOVABLE EQUIPMENT AND FURNITURE

Shower chairs
Portable hydraulic bath lift (stationary equipment preferred)
Bathroom safety devices
Hanging plants
Wastebasket

RELATIONSHIPS

Necessary to:	Resident rooms
	Nurses' station
Desirable to:	Janitor's closet
	Clean linen storage
Undesirable to:	Hazardous areas
	Public areas

BUILT-IN EQUIPMENT

Showers or tubs both equipped for handicapped use

Lavatory

Bathtub equipped with hydraulic lifting device or other safety equipment

Nurse-call signaling device

Shower and privacy curtains

Floor drain

Paper towel dispenser

Mirror

Toilet paper holder

Soap dispenser

Training toilet, one generally required on each floor or at each nurses' station, 3-foot clearance needed on three sides for a helper. Arm rest required on both sides of toilet bowl. Making this space private will aid in bowel and bladder training.

Storage cabinets

CLIMATE CONTROL

Temperature:	80°F
	Provide infrared heaters in the drying areas to prevent chilling
Humidity:	30 to 50%
Outside air:	Optional
Total air changes:	10 per hour
	All air exhausted directly to outdoors to remove high moisture content and odors
Pressure relationship:	Negative
	Avoid drafts at the floor

LIGHTING

Quantity:	30 footcandles
Type:	Fluorescent

ACOUSTICS

Bathrooms are generally very noisy because of the hard wall and floor surfaces. Using water-resistant acoustical panels for the ceiling is rec-ommended. Adjacent areas should be protected from sound generated in this space.

SPECIAL CONSIDERATIONS

- Layout must be designed to make it accessible to the handicapped and provide visual privacy from the corridor.
- Staff members should be able to give assistance, without getting themselves wet, to the residents who take showers.

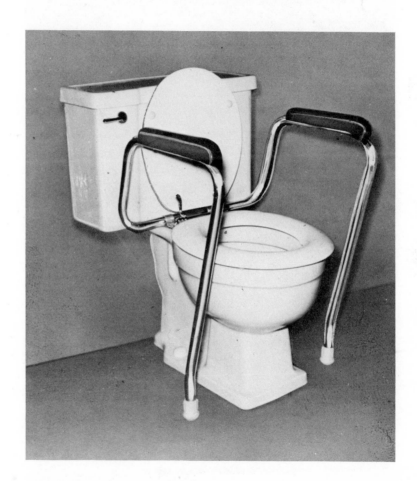

Training toilet using removeable floor-supported arm rest. (*Courtesy J. A. Preston Corporation*)

HEALTH AND PROFESSIONAL AREAS

Medical/Dental/Podiatry Area

This area should contain one or more treatment rooms and, if space permits, a private office for the physician and a waiting room. In a larger facility, a secretary may be needed to make appointments and to take care of the paperwork.

The residents have the option of using their own physician, but it generally evolves into having only a few physicians taking care of all the residents. A young doctor just starting out or an elderly person who is trying to slow down are the best candidates. Daily routine examinations are done in the residents' rooms. Minor examinations and treatments are done in the medical office, and, when indicated, residents are taken outside of the facility to the offices of the specialists. The physicians prefer this, and it gives the resident a chance to "go out."

The type of medicine practiced in a long-term care facility is the chronic type, not "acute." Most of the residents have long-term problems, and, in most cases, it is better to leave them in the facility rather than transfer them to a hospital. Moving an elderly person to a hospital is a traumatic experience, and most physicians will try to avoid it except in extreme cases. Recovery is more likely in familiar surroundings and in the company of friends; for this reason some intensive care type rooms should be maintained where a sick resident can be transferred.

ACTIVITIES

Examination and treatment in the following specialties:

> Dental
> Eye
> Ear, nose, throat
> General medical
> Podiatry

NUMBER OF USERS

3 people per office

PRIMARY USERS

Physicians and other professionals
Residents
Nursing personnel

SECONDARY USERS

Laboratory workers
Housekeeping workers
Maintenance workers

RELATIONSHIPS

Necessary to:	Toilet
	Storage closets
Desirable to:	Resident rooms
	Medical supply storage
	Administrative area
	Lobby
Undesirable to:	Hazardous areas

ATMOSPHERE

Cheerful
Healthy
Relaxed

COLOR SCHEME

Warm colors with bright accents

SPACE CONFIGURATION

Size:	1 or 2 offices: 120 to 150 square feet
	Reception or waiting area: 100 to 150 square feet
Ceiling height:	8 to 9 feet

INTERIOR SURFACES

Floor:	Easily maintained and cleaned
	Moisture proof
	Resilient
	Durable
	Non-slip
	Resilient tile
	Sheet vinyl
Walls:	Easily maintained and cleaned
	Washable within reach
	Vinyl wall covering
	Gypsum wallboard
Ceiling:	Acoustical treatment recommended
	Acoustical tile
	Gypsum wallboard

MOVABLE EQUIPMENT AND FURNITURE

Examining table
Desk
2 or 3 chairs
Wastebasket
Storage cabinets
Medical equipment

BUILT-IN EQUIPMENT

Lavatory
Dental chair, can double as podiatry and eye examination chair
Utility connections for equipment
Internal communication system

CLIMATE CONTROL

Temperature:	75°F
Humidity:	30 to 50%
Outside air:	2 air changes per hour
Total air changes:	6 per hour
Pressure relationship:	Negative

LIGHTING

General lighting should present a pleasing, relaxing atmostphere but should also produce a color consistent with proper diagnosis of a resident's condition. General lighting should be complemented with localized lighting for specific areas needing higher levels of illumination.

In addition to general lighting necessary for office type tasks, low level lighting should be provided which varies down to total darkness.

Quantity:	50 footcandles/general
	100 footcandles/detail
Type:	Fluorescent
	Incandescent
	Rheostat (dimmer) controlled lighting for eye examination is required. Light controls should be convenient to the physician.

ACOUSTICS

Adjacent area should be protected from sound generated in this space.

AUXILIARY SPACES

Toilet:
   Should open directly from the examination space and be accessible to the handicapped
Storage closets:
   Lockable storage space is required for medical supplies, instruments, equipment, etc.

Physical Therapy Room

The rehabilitation process centers mostly on helping the residents function as independently as possible and teaching them how to deal with their disabilities. The amount of equipment to be included in a facility will depend on the number and type of residents, the availability of treatment elsewhere, and the philosophy and budget of the administrative body.

In a 120-bed home, two part-time therapists will be able to handle the work load. A word of caution here: It is common to have too much

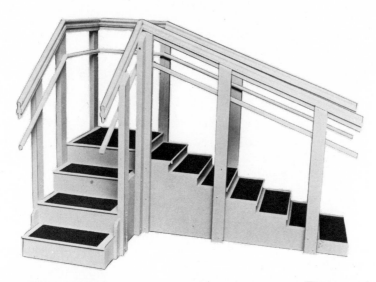

Corner-style exercise staircase. Four six-inch steps on one side, eight three-inch steps on the other. Steps are 36 inches wide. (*Courtesy of J. A. Preston Corporation*)

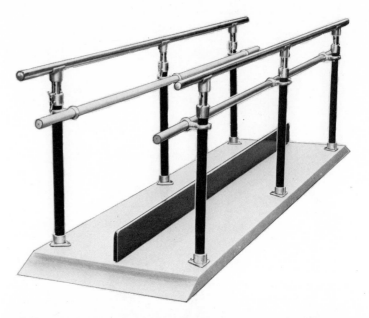

Walking parallel bars mounted on platform. Upper handrail adjustable, ten feet long; width between upper handrails is 24 inches. (*Courtesy J. A. Preston Corporation*)

equipment in the non-profit facilities and not enough in the proprietary ones. It is better to start out with minimum equipment as long as adequate space is provided, so that additional equipment can be accommodated later.

Physical therapy should not be limited to this designated room only. It should go on in the corridors (walking) and even in the residents' beds by using portable devices.

ACTIVITIES

Diagnostic work and testing
Ambulation
Therapeutic exercise
Electrotherapy and pain control
Heat and cold therapy
Hydrotherapy
Training in the use of independence aids
Massage

NUMBER OF USERS

4 to 6 residents
1 or 2 therapists or therapy assistants

PRIMARY USERS

Residents
Physical therapist
Therapy assistants

SECONDARY USERS

Nursing personnel
Volunteers (transportation only)
Physicians
Housekeeping workers
Maintenance workers

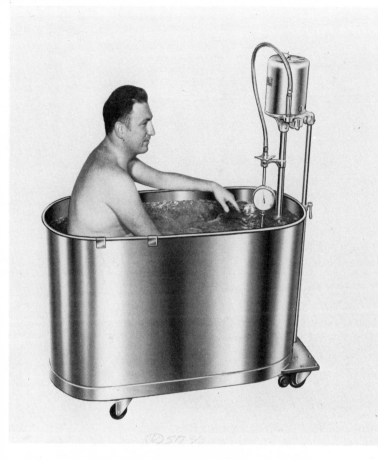

Mobile whirlpool bath. (*Courtesy of J. A. Preston Corporation*)

RELATIONSHIPS

Necessary to:	Toilet
	Storage
Desirable to:	Medical area
	Nurses' station
	Outdoor walking areas

ATMOSPHERE

Active	Stimulating
Cheerful	

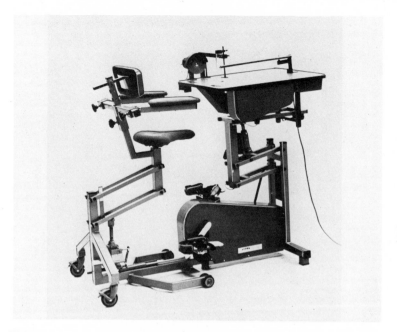

Therapeutic cycle. Totally adjustable machine to facilitate motion in various parts of the body. Operation of adjustable foot pedals activates the tools. (*Courtesy of J. A. Preston Corporation*)

COLOR SCHEME

Warm color range	Primary colors for accents

SPACE CONFIGURATION

Size:	Minimum 300 square feet
	Approximately 3 square feet per bed
Ceiling height:	8 to 10 feet

INTERIOR SURFACES

Floor:	Easily maintained and cleaned
	Moisture proof
	Resilient
	Durable
	Non-slip
	Resilient tile
	Sheet vinyl

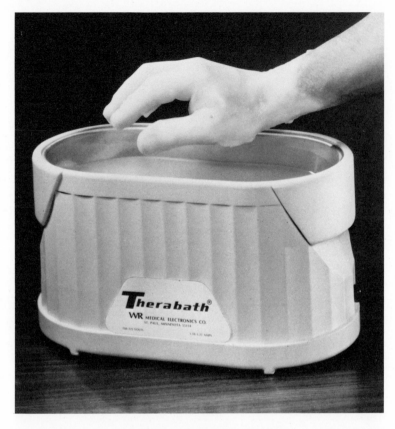

Paraffin bath. Effective method of applying heat uniformly for relief of pain. (*Courtesy of W. R. Medical Electronics Co.*)

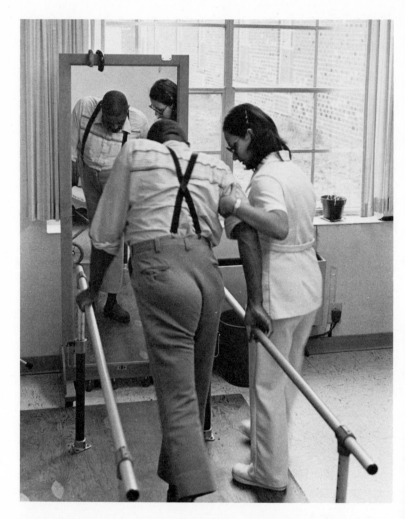

A stroke victim using parallel bars. Note the mirror which permits resident to observe his movements. (*Photographer: Bobby Thompson*)

Walls:	Easily maintained and cleaned
	Washable within reach
	Vinyl wall covering
	Ceramic tile
	Gypsum wallboard
Ceiling:	Acoustical treatment recommended
	Acoustical tile
	Gypsum wallboard

MOVABLE EQUIPMENT AND FURNITURE

Posture training mirrors
Walking parallel bars (adjustable width and height)
Walking aids (walkers, crutches, canes, quad canes, wheelchairs)
Exercise staircase (corner or straight type)

Raised exercise mats
Stationary bicycle exerciser
Overhead pulley weights
Shoulder wheel
Restorator (bicycle type portable equipment can be used in bed or sitting in a regular chair)
Ultrasound equipment
Electronic nerve stimulators
Electronic pain suppression equipment
Massage vibrators
Infra-red lamps
Ultra-violet lamps
Paraffin baths

Hot-pack unit
Cold-pack unit
Whirlpool baths
Traction equipment
Treatment tables (fixed or adjustable)
Tilt tables
Mirrors
Clock
Cubicle curtains

BUILT-IN EQUIPMENT

Cubicle curtain tracks
Lavatory
Whirlpool
Utility connections for portable and built-in equipment
Structural reinforcement required for ceiling or wall-mounted equipment
Internal communication system (telephone intercom or portable paging)

CLIMATE CONTROL

Temperature:	75°F
Humidity:	30 to 50%
Outside air:	2 air changes per hour
Total air changes:	6 per hour
Pressure relationship:	Negative

LIGHTING

Quantity:	30 footcandles/general
Type:	Fluorescent

ACOUSTICS

Adjacent areas should be protected from sound generated in this space.

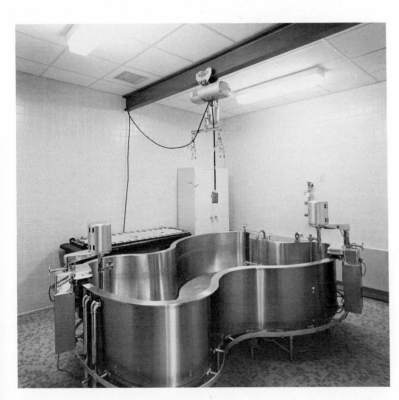

Full body immersion tank. (Daughters of Sarah Nursing Home, Albany, N. Y.; Donald J. Stephens Associates, Architect)

SPECIAL CONSIDERATIONS

Outdoor hard surfaced walking areas equipped with handrail (at least on one side) should be provided nearby. Surface material to be smooth but should not become slippery when wet.

AUXILIARY SPACES

Storage room: This room is required to store the following:

> Clean linen
> Towels
> Walkers
> Canes
> Crutches
> Wheelchairs
> Other miscellaneous supplies and
> devices

Size:	80 to 120 square feet
Built-in equipment:	Shelving
Lighting:	30 footcandles
	Fluorescent

Office for physical therapist: This may be just an area within the physical therapy room but a private office is preferred.

> Movable equipment or furniture
> Filing cabinets
> Desk with drawers
> 3 chairs
> Bulletin board
> Chalk board
> Telephone
> Additional requirements for this room are similar to other professional offices

Toilet for residents: Provide sufficient room around toilet bowl for toilet training (learning how to get on and off). See Toilets (for resident rooms) for detailed description of other requirements.

Speech Therapy Room

Many residents who require speech therapy can be treated at bedside, but there is the problem of the resident being distracted and the inconvenience of transporting the equipment used in the therapy. A small room would solve these and other problems related to speech therapy.

ACTIVITIES

Diagnostic work and testing
Retraining

NUMBER OF USERS

2 to 3 people

PRIMARY USERS

Residents
Therapists

SECONDARY USERS

Nursing personnel
Volunteers
Housekeeping workers
Maintenance workers

RELATIONSHIPS

Necessary to:	Toilet
Desirable to:	Resident rooms
Undesirable to:	Noisy areas

ATMOSPHERE

Calm, quiet
Absence of audible and visible distractions

COLOR SCHEME

Cool colors

Size:	150 to 180 square feet
Ceiling height:	8 to 10 feet

INTERIOR SURFACES

Floor:
Easily maintained and cleaned
Moisture proof
Resilient
Resilient tile
Sheet vinyl

Walls:
Easily maintained and cleaned
Gypsum wallboard
Vinyl wall covering

Ceiling:
Acoustical treatment recommended
Acoustical tile
Gypsum wallboard

MOVABLE EQUIPMENT AND FURNITURE

Desk with file drawers
3 chairs
Credenza or small storage cabinet
Table (high enough for use by a wheelchair-bound resident)
Tape recorder
Language master (a tabletop teaching aid)
Mirror

BUILT-IN EQUIPMENT

Internal communication system

CLIMATE CONTROL

Temperature:	75°F
Humidity:	30 to 50%
Outside air:	2 air changes per hour
Total air changes:	6 per hour
Pressure relationship:	Equal

LIGHTING

Quantity:	30 footcandles/general
	70 footcandles/detail
Type:	Fluorescent

ACOUSTICS

Complete acoustical separation must be maintained.

Social Worker's Office

The social worker's activities in a long-term care facility include interviewing prospective residents to ascertain whether or not the facility and staff can meet the social needs of the person, gathering social histories of residents, counseling with residents and their families, documenting the resident's social progress and frequently shopping for the resident or at least delegating that responsibility to someone else. The social worker is sometimes faced with the necessity of dealing with a family's guilt feelings. This was a larger problem in years past, but, with the acceptance of long-term care facilities as a viable and often preferable alternative to home care, the incidence of guilt has diminished.

The social worker may be an invaluable person in staff education regarding the psycho-social needs of older people, their perceptual and sensory deprivations and the wide range of experience in a long-term care facility which encompasses the social component of care. The social worker as a skilled counselor can effectively intercede in the resolution of staff personal problems which may cause excessive absenteeism, tardiness, poor work habits, etc.

ACTIVITIES

Counseling or interviewing residents or prospective residents, their families or responsible parties
Writing social histories and progress notes on residents
Admission work

NUMBER OF USERS

1 to 5

PRIMARY USERS

Social worker
Residents
Family members of residents

SECONDARY USERS

Other social workers
Other department heads
Housekeeping workers
Maintenance workers

RELATIONSHIPS

Necessary to:	Resident areas
Desirable to:	Offices of director of nurses
	Activity director
	Administrative offices
	Lobby
Undesirable to:	Kitchen
	Laundry

ATMOSPHERE

Quiet
Calm
Friendly
Relaxed

COLOR SCHEME

Warm color range
Pastel colors

SPACE CONFIGURATIONS

Size:	150 to 180 square feet
Ceiling height:	8 to 9 feet

INTERIOR SURFACES

Floor:	Resilient
	Easily maintained and cleaned
	Resilient tile
	Sheet vinyl
	Carpet
Walls:	Easily maintained and cleaned
	Vinyl wall covering
	Gypsum wallboard
Ceiling:	Acoustical treatment recommended
	Acoustical tile

MOVABLE EQUIPMENT AND FURNITURE

Desk with drawers
Filing cabinet
Typewriter
Telephone (with privacy button to prevent eavesdropping by others)
3 to 4 chairs
Book shelves
Credenza or cabinet

BUILT-IN EQUIPMENT

Internal communication system

CLIMATE CONTROL

Temperature:	75°F
Humidity:	30 to 50%
Outside air:	7.5 cubic feet per minute per occupant
Total air changes:	6 per hour
Pressure relationship:	Equal

LIGHTING

Quantity:	30 footcandles/general
	70 footcandles/detail
Type:	Fluorescent or incandescent

Sound privacy is a must since the discussions between residents, family members, and social worker will be of a confidential nature.

SPECIAL CONSIDERATION

If space permits an additional office should be provided for social work students. Schools are always trying to place their students in order to fulfill their "practicum" requirements. The facility and the school will both benefit from an arrangement like this; however, in this case there should be a supervisor with an M.S.W. (Masters of Social Work) degree on the staff.

Office of the Director of Nursing

The Director of Nursing has the overall responsibility for all the nursing care and is one of the key persons in deciding if a person will be admitted. This person is in charge of organizing all the medically oriented activities, seeing to it that: the physician's orders are carried out; medications administered; laboratory tests are done and recorded; and examinations are carried out. The actual nursing is done by the "charge nurse" at the nursing unit and the aides and orderlies.

ACTIVITIES

Speaking to residents
Meeting with staff members
Consulting with families of residents
Organizing nursing care
Administrative work

NUMBER OF USERS

2 to 4 people

PRIMARY USER

Director of Nursing

SECONDARY USERS

Assistant Director of Nursing
Nursing personnel
Residents
Families of residents
Other department heads
Housekeeping workers
Maintenance workers

RELATIONSHIPS

Necessary to:	Nurses' stations
	Office of the Assistant Director of Nursing
Desirable to:	Medical supply storage
	Administrative offices
	Toilet

ATMOSPHERE

Quiet
Calm
Friendly
Relaxed

COLOR SCHEME

Pastel colors

SPACE CONFIGURATION

Size:	120 to 150 square feet
Ceiling height:	8 to 9 feet

INTERIOR SURFACES

Floor:	Resilient
	Easily maintained and cleaned
	Resilient tile
	Sheet vinyl
	Carpet

Walls:	Easily maintained and cleaned
	Vinyl wall covering
	Gypsum wallboard
Ceiling:	Acoustical treatment recommended
	Acoustical tile

MOVABLE EQUIPMENT AND FURNITURE

Desk with drawers	Book shelves
3 to 4 chairs	Telephone
Filing cabinets	Wastebasket

BUILT-IN EQUIPMENT

Internal communication system

CLIMATE CONTROL

Temperature:	70° to 75°F
Humidity:	30 to 50%
Outside air:	7.5 cubic feet per minute per occupant
Total air changes:	6 per hour
Pressure relationship:	Equal

LIGHTING

Quantity:	30 footcandles/general
	70 footcandles/detail
Type:	Fluorescent

ACOUSTICS

Maintain acoustical privacy in this room, many of the discussions will be confidential.

AUXILIARY SPACES

Office of the Assistant Director of Nursing: In larger facilities an assistant may be required. This office should be adjacent to the office of the director of nursing. All other requirements should be identical except that it should be smaller for ''political'' reasons.

Pharmacy

A 120-bed long-term care facility is not sufficiently large to support an in-house pharmacy. However, occasionally a retired pharmacist wishing to keep active may want to establish a pharmacy within a facility. There are some advantages to be gained by this arrangement, as long as the pharmacist is willing to make himself readily available. Pharmacy laws vary from state-to-state, but most states limit access into the pharmacy to the pharmacists or their assistants. Therefore having a pharmacy located on premises does not necessarily mean that a needed drug will be readily available; the pharmacist must be there to personally dispense the drug. It is possible, too, that an enterprising pharmacist may use this facility as a base from which to serve other clients.

ACTIVITIES

Preparing and dispensing of medications

NUMBER OF USERS

1 to 2 people

PRIMARY USER

Pharmacist

SECONDARY USERS

Pharmacy technician
Delivery personnel
Pharmaceutical company representatives

RELATIONSHIPS

Necessary to:	Receiving area
Desirable to:	Nurses' stations
Undesirable to:	Any area not well supervised

ATMOSPHERE

Simple
Businesslike

SPACE CONFIGURATION

Size: 300 square feet minimum

Ceiling height: 8 to 10 feet

INTERIOR SURFACES

Floor: Easily maintained and cleaned
                               Resilient tile
                               Sheet vinyl

Walls: Gypsum wallboard
                               Masonry

Ceiling: Gypsum wallboard

MOVABLE EQUIPMENT AND FURNITURE

Pharmacy ''Rules and Regulations'' should be consulted for specifics but generally some movable and fixed shelving, a typewriter, prescription balances, a refrigerator and the usual accouterments required by the profession.

BUILT-IN EQUIPMENT

Sink
Shelving
Countertop—about 10 to 12 feet by 2 feet
Cabinets
Safe (may be required for storage of some drugs)
An alarm device is frequently required by law
Internal communication system

CLIMATE CONTROL

Temperature: 75°F
Humidity: 30 to 50%
Outside air: 2 air changes
Total air changes: 4 per hour
Pressure relationship: Positive

LIGHTING

Quantity: 30 footcandles/general
                               70 footcandles/detail
Type: Fluorescent

SPECIAL CONSIDERATIONS

- Extra caution must be exercised to minimize the possibility of drug losses by preventing unauthorized entry through doors, walls and ceiling. The door should not be openable by a master key.
- A Dutch door through which drug orders could be passed would be useful.

Medical Supply Room

This room is used for bulk storage of medical and nursing supplies, such as medicine cups, parenteral solutions, bulk drugs i.e. milk of magnesia, mineral oil, hydrogen peroxide, etc. The items stored in this room will be expensive; therefore, security must be good. Adjustable shelving must be provided, so that the items can be arranged in an orderly fashion. Disarray in this room will surely result in some items being overstocked and other items being out of stock which could jeopardize the well-being of some residents.

NUMBER OF USERS

2 to 3 people

PRIMARY USERS

Nursing personnel

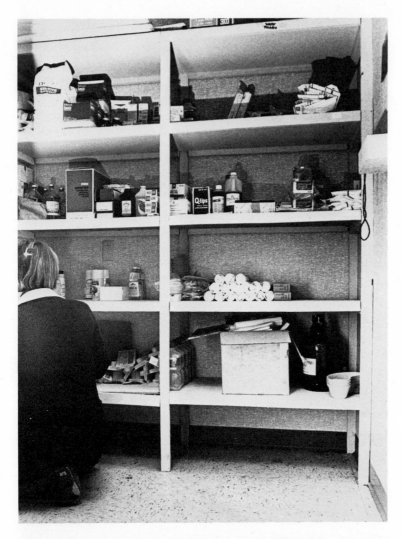

Medical supply room. Simple fixed wood shelving is adequate, but adjustable shelving is better because of the greater flexibility provided. (*Photographer: Bobby Thompson*)

SECONDARY USERS

Medical/nursing supply sales representatives
Housekeeping workers
Maintenance workers

RELATIONSHIPS

Necessary to:	Nurses' stations
Desirable to:	Receiving area
Undesirable to:	Low security areas

SPACE CONFIGURATION

Size:	150 to 200 square feet
	Room will be needed to maneuver large cartons on a hand truck.
Ceiling height:	8 to 10 feet

INTERIOR SURFACES

Floor:	Resilient tile
	Painted concrete
Walls:	Gypsum wallboard
	Masonry
Ceiling:	Gypsum wallboard
	Acoustical tile

BUILT-IN EQUIPMENT

150 to 200 linear feet of 18-inch deep shelving
Desk or counter for the purpose of charging out supplies

CLIMATE CONTROL

Temperature:	75°F
Humidity:	30 to 50%
Outside air:	2 air changes per hour
Total air changes:	4 per hour
Pressure relationship:	Positive

LIGHTING

Quantity:	30 footcandles
Type:	Fluorescent

Security may be a problem. Measures should be taken to prevent unauthorized entry through doors, walls and ceiling. If acoustical tile ceiling is used surrounding walls should extend to structure above for security.

Medical Record Room

The data found in a resident's chart is no longer limited to medical information. Charts now include social histories, overall care plans, discharge plans, etc. The chart is kept at the nurses' station, accessible to nursing and other professionals. Because of the amount of data inputted daily, the charts must be culled frequently. Some long-staying residents' records will have to be moved because of the sheer volume to the medical record storage. The records of discharged (to home, to another facility or by death) Medicaid residents must be retained in accordance with State law. However, if there is no State law, records must still be retained for five years after discharge of a skilled care, Medicaid resident or three years after discharge of an intermediate care, Medicaid resident. Record retention requirements make storage at the nurses' station impractical. Typically, the current charts will be at the nurses' station. The culled records of residents who are still in the facility will be stored in the office of the Director of Nursing. The records of discharged residents will be stored elsewhere in the facility in the Medical Record Room. Some facilities have turned to microfilming as a solution to the mounting problem of record storage.

NUMBER OF USERS

2 to 3 people

PRIMARY USERS

Director of Nursing
Social worker
Activity Director

SECONDARY USERS

Housekeeping workers
Maintenance workers

RELATIONSHIPS

Desirable to: Administrative area
Office of the Director of Nursing

SPACE CONFIGURATION

Size: 150 to 200 square feet
Ceiling height: 8 feet

INTERIOR SURFACES

There are no special requirements; however, at least one hour fire rated construction recommended for the protection of the records.

MOVABLE EQUIPMENT AND FURNITURE

Filing cabinets (both legal and letter size)

LIGHTING

Quantity: 50 footcandles
Type: Fluorescent

SPECIAL CONSIDERATIONS

Medical records are of confidential nature. The access to this area should be limited to authorized persons only. This must be considered when the keying system is designed.

Staff Development Room

Formerly and still frequently called in-service training, staff development differs from the latter term only in the respect that it is more comprehensive. Each facility should develop a curriculum dealing with all aspects of operating a long-term care facility. The curriculum would be the result of input from the various disciplines. Most of the course material will be delivered on-premises by staff people, but some of the material will necessarily be offered outside the facility and delivered by other professionals. The important point is that the curriculum be well thought out, comprehensive, timely and committed to paper. Furthermore, it is essential that good attendance records be maintained. It should be possible, for example, to know where any particular worker stands, with respect to completing the course material for his job, by referring to his personnel folder. The curriculum must allow for some flexibility, for changes in course material, inclusion of new material and for changes in personnel delivering the material.

Several companies produce films, slides, film strips and other aides for effective delivery of course material. Housekeeping supply distributors, equipment manufacturers or distributors, pharmacies or pharmaceutical manufacturers, etc. often have excellent educational materials and are willing to provide training sessions.

Staff development should contain something for every worker from the administrator on down. Program administration should rest with a single individual, who must be thought of as the "headmaster." Recognition should be given to any individual who has completed the course material in his discipline. Such recognition need not be more than a certificate. This is so simple as to seem unimportant. Remember that most of the facility's workers will be minimum wage people, who have had only minimum education and to them recognition is important.

Staff development takes place in many different areas within the building. Staff development for dietary workers most frequently is delivered in the kitchen. Other locations would include the resident's room, the laundry or the corridors. When larger groups are assembled, the dining room, the activity room or the conference room may be used. A room may be set aside exclusively for staff development. In that case, the specific requirements for the room will be very similar to the conference room.

Morgue

Some facilities provide a morgue. It should be pointed out that more often than not the resident dies in the hospital or in an intensive care unit room within the facility, where he would have been transferred at the onset of an acute illness. An alternative to a morgue is to draw the cubicle curtain around the bed in multi-bedded rooms until the body can be moved. Of course, there is no problem in a single-bedded room. Should a morgue be found desirable, it should be a room large enough to accommodate a stretcher (about 30 inches by 74 inches) and located near an exit leading to a driveway. A room 50 to 60 square feet appears to be adequate.

84

Outside air:	Optional
Total air changes:	10 per hour
Pressure relationship:	Negative

LIGHTING

Quantity:	20 footcandles
Type:	Fluorescent

FOOD SERVICE AREAS

Kitchen

No attempt will be made here to produce a complete list of equipment to furnish a kitchen. Ordinarily, the designer will seek assistance in equipping and laying out the kitchen. Unfortunately he oftentimes finds that the only assistance available is from a kitchen-supply company which, of course, is in business to sell equipment. Is there a solution to this dilemma? No easy one. It would be best for the designer or owner to educate himself enough to be a little more than conversant relative to the kitchen, then to seek advice from the supplier, a dietitian, a state official in another state who oversees kitchen construction (no axe to grind), dietary workers and finally other long-term care facility operators. Remember the various points of view involved. The dietitian, dietary worker and facility operator will be most concerned with functional considerations; the supplier with making the sale; and the State with meeting standards, and the latter will sometimes attempt to force higher than official standards on the owner. A kitchen design consultant, if he has no "ties" to a manufacturer, can be a valuable aide in solving this very important problem.

The way food is to be served will impact on the design. Food may be served on plates or segmented trays. Residents may be served in the dining rooms, but some, because of their condition, will be served in their rooms. Food will have to be transported from the kitchen to the dining rooms or to the residents' rooms. If this be the case, the designer must determine the number of carts needed and where such carts will be stored within the kitchen area when not in use. In contrast, if most residents will be served in a central dining room, fewer

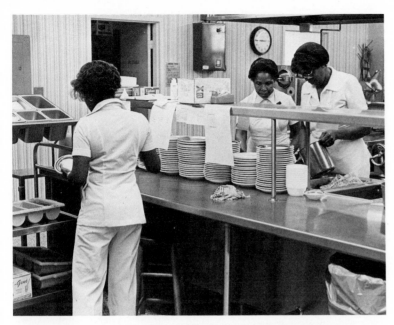

Dietary workers preparing the evening meal. To the left of the clock is the manual control for the range hood fire extinguishing system. (Health Care Center of Raleigh, Raleigh, N.C.; *Photographer: Bobby Thompson*)

or no carts will be needed. It is the owner who, after due consideration of the various points of view, must decide the kind of food service to be offered, before the kitchen design consultant can begin his planning.

In keeping with the philosophy of this book, food served on plates is recommended. Plated-food may be placed on a tray and the tray in a cart for transportation to the resident. If the food must be served in the resident's room, or in a remote dining room, then adequate measures must be taken to assure that the food will be hot when served. In fact, standards require that any perishable food or ingredient capable of supporting rapid growth of harmful organisms must be maintained at safe temperatures; that is, at 45°F or below or 140°F or above from the time of preparation, until it is served to the resident. This can be accomplished in several ways. The two most widely used methods are the use of a heated cart for transportation or the use of a heated plate liner; the cart is heated electrically in the kitchen prior to loading; the plate liner is heated in a heater stationed in the kitchen. Unless handled with care, these liners can cause burns.

Newer food service systems employ elaborate carts, make wide use of disposables, and their promoters claim reduced man-hours of labor. While the disposables are attractively made, they still appear institutional. Improvements in these systems will be forthcoming, and the designer and owner should consider this option carefully. There are several organizations which now offer contract dietary service. Food may be prepared on premises or off-premises, as would be done for airlines.

ACTIVITIES

Cooking
Baking
Plate preparation
Cleaning

NUMBER OF USERS

8 to 12 people

PRIMARY USERS

Dietary supervisor
Cooks
Dietary aides

SECONDARY USERS

Delivery people
Sales people
Equipment repairmen
Maintenance workers

RELATIONSHIPS

Necessary to:

Dining room
Dietary supervisor's office
Dry storage
Refrigerated storage
Freezers
Loading area

Desirable to:	Toilets
	Staff lockers
	Refuse disposal area
	Can washing room
	Staff dining room
	Boiler room
Undesirable to:	Resident rooms
	Administrative areas
	Lobby

SPACE CONFIGURATION

| Size: | 1200 to 1500 square feet |
| Ceiling height: | 10 to 12 feet |

INTERIOR SURFACES

Floors:	Easily maintained and cleaned
	Moisture proof
	Non-slip
	Quarry tile with acid resistant grout
Walls:	Easily maintained and cleaned
	Ceramic tile
Ceiling:	Moisture proof
	Plaster
	Acoustical tile (moisture proof)

MOVABLE EQUIPMENT AND FURNITURE

Cooking utensils
Dishes
Silverware
Carts
Tray trucks
Shelving
Trash receptacles
Clock

BUILT-IN EQUIPMENT

Consult a specialist in this field for detailed requirements. The following is a representative list of equipment usually found in a long-term care facility, some of these items could be movable or built-in:

Beverage stand
Coffee urn
Water station with ice bin
Glass and cup racks
Instant iced tea dispenser
Tray rest with china storage
Roll warmer
Cook's table with hot food unit
Canopy with lights, filter, exhaust fan
Convection oven
Steamer
Steam kettle
Tilting skillet
Fryer
Griddle-top range
Utensil rack
Potato peeler
Vegetable sink with disposer
Slicer
Work tables
Mixer
Baker's table with portable ingredient bins
Ice machine
Soiled dish table
Booster heater
Disposal unit
Pre-wash sink
Dish washing machine
Clean dish table
Utensil sink with drain board
Shelving
Refrigerator
Walk-in refrigerator
Freezer
Walk-in freezer
Ice cream cabinet
Lavatory

CLIMATE CONTROL

Temperature: 75°F
Outside air: 2 air changes per hour
Total air changes: 10 per hour
Pressure relationship: Negative
                              All air exhausted directly to the outside.
                              Note: Air conditioning is not customary.

LIGHTING

Quantity: 70 footcandles
Type: Fluorescent
                Mercury vapor
                Incandescent

ACOUSTICS

The kitchen generally is a noisy place. Noise should be controlled internally and steps should be taken to minimize the noise transfer to adjacent spaces, particularly into the dining room.

SPECIAL CONSIDERATION

There may be special dietary consideration in a particular facility. Jewish homes generally require a kosher kitchen, with some or all the equipment duplicated in two separate kitchens, dairy and meat products being separated.

AUXILIARY SPACES

Janitor's closet: Storage for housekeeping equipment and supplies. Provide floor receptor or service sink.

Waste storage room: This room must be easily accessible to the outside for pickup or disposal. All air from this room should be exhausted directly to outdoors.

Can washing room: Provide floor receptor or drain, hot and cold water faucet. Wall and floor surfaces to be easily cleanable. All air from this room should be exhausted directly to outdoors.

Dietary Supervisor's Office

State regulations require that a staff member who is qualified by education or training in food management be designated as the dietary (or food service) supervisor. This person is responsible for planning menus, purchasing food and supervising the preparation of the food, including therapeutic diets. A small office will be required next to the kitchen with good visibility into the kitchen. Most states require the services of a consulting certified dietitian to assist with the food service planning and in-service education.

ACTIVITIES

Menu planning
Food and dietary supply ordering
Interviewing of workers

NUMBER OF USERS

1 or 2 people

PRIMARY USER

Dietary supervisor

SECONDARY USERS

Dietary workers
Salespersons
Consultant dietitian
Maintenance workers

RELATIONSHIPS

Necessary to: Kitchen
                       Kitchen storage

Desirable to: Toilet

SPACE CONFIGURATION

Size: 80 to 100 square feet
Ceiling height: 8 feet

Floor:	Resilient tile
Walls:	Any painted surface
Ceiling:	Acoustical tile
	Gypsum wallboard

MOVABLE EQUIPMENT AND FURNITURE

Desk
2 or 3 chairs
Filing cabinet
Calculator
Wastebasket
Bulletin board

BUILT-IN EQUIPMENT

Telephone
Internal communication system
Observation windows

CLIMATE CONTROL

Temperature:	75°F
Humidity:	30 to 50%
Outside air:	7.5 cubic feet per minute
Total air changes:	6 per hour
Pressure relationship:	Positive

LIGHTING

Quantity:	30 footcandles/general
	70 footcandles/detail
Type:	Fluorescent

ACOUSTICS

Acoustical privacy should be maintained. Some transactions may be confidential.

88

SPECIAL CONSIDERATION

The dietary supervisor must insure against pilferage, and for that reason this person's office is best placed where close supervision of the workers is possible.

Kitchen Storage

Kitchen storage includes refrigerated and dry storage. A 120-bed facility is large enough to make a walk-in freezer and walk-in refrigerator of modest size economically feasible. This would meet only a part of the cold storage requirements; smaller refrigerators and freezers meet daily requirements. The total of all cold storage requirements will be about 2 cubic feet per bed. Most other foods, condiments and usually some paper products, will be stored in the dry storage area, which will be the subject of this section. Both cold and dry storage areas must be big enough for the dietary supervisor to store foods acquired in bulk when prices are low, but not so large as to encourage overpurchasing, which will result in loss from spoilage.

ACTIVITIES

Storing of foods and supplies
Inventorying of foods and supplies
Retrieving of foods and supplies

NUMBER OF USERS

2 to 3 people

PRIMARY USERS

Dietary supervisor
Dietary workers

SECONDARY USERS

Salespersons
Maintenance workers

Necessary to: Kitchen
Desirable to: Receiving area

SPACE CONFIGURATION

Size: 200 to 250 square feet
Ceiling height: 8 to 10 feet

INTERIOR SURFACES

Floor: Easily maintained and cleaned
                  Moisture proof
                  Quarry tile
                  Sealed concrete

Walls: Easily maintained and cleaned
                  Gypsum wallboard
                  Masonry

Ceiling: Gypsm wallboard
                  Acoustical ceiling is acceptable only (because of security problems) when the surrounding walls are sealed against the structure above to prevent unauthorized entry.

MOVABLE EQUIPMENT AND FURNITURE

Adjustable stainless steel shelving preferred over painted, built-in, wood shelving. Movable shelving on wheels helps to keep the room clean.

CLIMATE CONTROL

Outside air: Optional
Total air changes: 2 per hour
Pressure relationship: Equal

LIGHTING

Quantity: 20 footcandles
Type: Fluorescent

SPECIAL CONSIDERATIONS

This area should be located to allow maximum supervision in order to discourage pilferage. Dietary supervisors should open this room only long enough to take out the items required to prepare the next meal. Measures should be taken to prevent unauthorized entry through doors, walls and ceiling.

Dining Room

The dining rooms of most long-term care facilities are offensive because of their strong institutional appearance. Dining rooms can be designed which are aesthetically pleasing but, at the same time, meet the need of being easily cleanable. A resident may spend years eating in that same dining room; it should be a pleasant experience. It should be noted that eating times are much anticipated events in the lives of the residents. It is also a time for socializing. Socialization is a normalizing experience that can be promoted by good design. Tables that seat four to six people encourage conversation. The use of low dividers, partitions and/or planters create intimate spaces. The architect should not forget everything he learned when he designed the town's most popular restaurant.

As an alternative, the designer might consider decentralized dining rooms. Such dining areas would likely be located within a nursing wing or even on different floors and would thereby greatly reduce the need for transporting the residents. These areas, because of the smaller size, would be more intimate and, being away from the kitchen, would likely be quieter; intimate and quiet dining promote socializing.

Decentralized dining rooms will necessitate the use of conveyors, dumb-waiters, food carts, etc. The resident's tray will be prepared in the kitchen, covered and slipped into a heated food cart. When full, the cart is transported to the remote dining area, where aides remove the trays to the tables. After the meal the trays are returned to the cart, which, in turn, is returned to the dishwashing area.

Some residents will require assistance with eating. That assistance might be given by an aide or a self-help device may be employed. These residents might create unsightly mess. The designer's problem will be to screen rather than isolate those individuals.

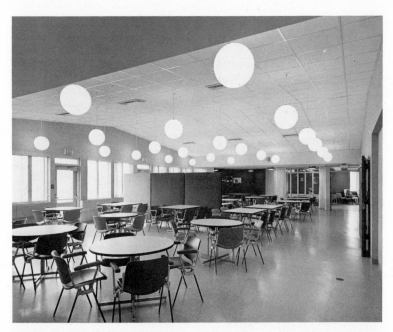

Sloping ceiling and hanging light fixtures tend to minimize the institutional feeling. Movable partitions separate the "hard to feed" residents. (*Daughters of Sarah Nursing Home, Albany, N. Y.; Donald J. Stephens Associates, Architects*)

The dietary supervisors of some facilities make it a policy to open the dining room doors only on a rigid schedule. Residents tend to congregate outside the dining room before meals, creating a congestion problem. The designer is wise to plan for this and provide adequate space in front of the dining room, which could well be another good socializing experience for the residents.

Serving buffet-style is worthy of consideration. It returns a measure of independence to the resident, who is able to make a choice, and it will not necessarily increase the cost of food service. If buffet-style serving is not feasible, a sense of independence, to a limited extent, can be achieved by providing the resident with an opportunity to toast bread, prepare a salad or pour his beverage.

Some facilities provide, adjacent to the dining room, a small "cocktail" lounge. While some will find the idea of serving residents alcoholic beverages abhorrent, even damaging, the reader must remember that he himself may someday be a resident of such a facility, and if a glass of wine before dinner has been a pleasant tradition, the denial of that may be a denial of his rights. Of course, the resident's physician should be consulted beforehand. In some states alcoholic beverages must be "prescribed" by a physician.

ACTIVITIES

Eating
Socializing
Special programs or performances
  See Activity Room for listing of other possible activities.

NUMBER OF USERS

80 to 90% of the residents plus dietary workers, altogether about 115 people

PRIMARY USERS

Residents
Dietary workers
Aides
Orderlies

SECONDARY USERS

Volunteers
Outside performing groups
Housekeeping workers
Maintenance workers

RELATIONSHIPS

Necessary to:	Kitchen
	Toilets
	Corridors
Desirable to:	Resident rooms
	Outdoors
Undesirable to:	Administrative areas
	Lobby
	Hazardous areas

ATMOSPHERE

Active
Stimulating
Restaurant-like

COLOR SCHEME

Warm color range
Primary accent colors

SPACE CONFIGURATION

Size: 15 square feet per user
                          Provide adequate aisle space for
                          wheelchair users

Ceiling height: 10 to 14 feet

INTERIOR SURFACES

Floor: Easily maintained and cleaned
                          Moisture proof
                          Resilient
                          Durable
                          Non-slip
                              Resilient tile
                              Sheet vinyl

Walls: Easily maintained and cleaned
                          Washable within reach
                              Vinyl wall covering
                              Gypsum wallboard

Ceiling: Acoustical treatment recommended
                              Acoustical tile
                              Gypsum wallboard

MOVABLE EQUIPMENT AND FURNITURE

Chairs
Tables (high enough for wheelchairs to fit under the tabletop, need
    about 30 inches clear)
Movable dividers
Paintings or pictures
Plants
Clock

BUILT-IN EQUIPMENT

Fireplace
Sound system

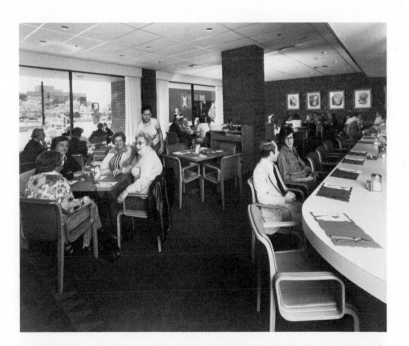

A view of the coffee shop at the newly completed Palisade Nursing Home in Riverdale. Here the residents can mingle with staff, board members or visitors. The coffee shop and an adjacent lounge area double as a "nightclub", where elderly residents can buy drinks and entertain friends and relatives. (Gruzen and Partners, Architects/Engineers; Photographer: Nathaniel Lieberman)

Temperature:	75° to 80°F
Humidity:	30 to 50%
Outside air:	4 air changes per hour
Total air changes:	6 per hour
Pressure relationship:	Equal

LIGHTING

Quantity:	30 footcandles
Type:	Incandescent
	Fluorescent
	Mercury vapor

Hanging light fixtures or chandeliers give a restaurant-like atmosphere.

Theater-type lighting may be required if live performances are contemplated.

ACOUSTICS

Acoustical treatment recommended to control internal noise and noise transfer to and from adjacent spaces.

SPECIAL CONSIDERATION

In some facilities the dining room doubles as the activity room. It is strongly recommended that separate spaces be provided, otherwise the activity-recreation functions will greatly suffer.

Staff Dining Room

The staff may dine in the main dining room after the residents have eaten or a separate staff dining room may be provided. This room might also serve food to visitors and be used as a staff meeting room or staff lounge between meals.

The governing body of the facility will have to make the determination whether the employees will be provided with food or not, and if they will have to pay for it. This will also depend on the neighborhood. If there are a great number of eating establishments within walking distance, a staff dining room may not be necessary. However, in many cases the long-term care facility will be in a remote area, requiring food service for the employees. There is still a problem how to provide for the night shift when the kitchen is closed. The usual solution is to provide vending machines for hot and cold food and drinks.

ACTIVITIES

Eating
Socializing
Staff meeting

NUMBER OF USERS

30 to 40 people

PRIMARY USERS

Staff members

SECONDARY USERS

Volunteers
Visitors
Housekeeping workers
Maintenance workers

RELATIONSHIPS

Necessary to:	Kitchen
Desirable to:	Staff lockers
	Toilets
	Service entrance
Undesirable to:	Resident areas

ATMOSPHERE

Cheerful
Relaxed

COLOR SCHEME

Pastel colors

SPACE CONFIGURATION

Size: 350 to 450 square feet
Ceiling height: 8 to 10 feet

INTERIOR SURFACES

Floor:
Easily maintained and cleaned
Moisture proof
Resilient
Durable
Non-slip
    Resilient tile
    Sheet vinyl

Walls:
Easily maintained and cleaned
Washable within reach
    Vinyl wall covering
    Gypsum wallboard

Ceiling:
Acoustical treatment recommended
    Acoustical tile
    Gypsum wallboard

MOVABLE EQUIPMENT AND FURNITURE

Tables
Chairs
Refrigerator
Microwave oven
Coffee maker
Waste baskets
Clock
Plants
Vending machines

BUILT-IN EQUIPMENT

Cafeteria style food service equipment, unless food is served directly from the kitchen.

CLIMATE CONTROL

Temperature: 75°F
Humidity: 30 to 50%
Outside air: 4 air changes per hour
Total air changes: 6 per hour
Pressure relationship: Equal

LIGHTING

Quantity: 30 footcandles
Type: Fluorescent

ACOUSTICS

Adjacent areas should be protected from sound generated in this space.

ADMINISTRATIVE AREAS

Lobby

It is often heard that there is no second chance to create a first impression. For this reason the treatment of this space is vitally important. In many instances, people have terrible guilt feelings about placing their parents in an "institution." A drab, cold, institutional lobby will only increase this guilt. The lobby usually serves as the main entrance for employees, visitors, prospective residents and their families, local, state and federal regulatory agents. It sometimes becomes a lounge for residents; however, this should be discouraged. An incontinent resident can turn an otherwise pleasant lobby into a "turn off" in a matter of minutes. An information area should be located here for the greeting of visitors and to provide security. The person providing this service could be a staff member or a volunteer. In larger facilities a separate reception area may be provided.

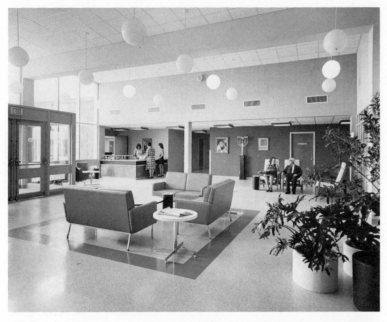

Spacious, well lit entrance area. Note presence of reception desk to provide security. (*Daughters of Sarah Nursing Home, Albany, N. Y.; Donald J. Stephens Associates, Architects*)

NUMBER OF USERS

10 to 15 people

PRIMARY USERS

All employees (unless another entrance is provided for their use)

SECONDARY USERS

Visitors	Volunteers
Residents	Housekeeping workers
Prospective residents	Maintenance workers
Families of residents	
Regulatory agents	
Salespeople	
Physicians	

RELATIONSHIPS

Necessary to:	Covered entrance area
	Parking
Desirable to:	Administrative area
	Public toilets
	Volunteer lounge
	Social worker's office
Undesirable to:	Resident areas
	Hazardous areas

ATMOSPHERE

Warm
Welcoming
Comfortable
Residential

COLOR SCHEME

Warm colors

SPACE CONFIGURATION

Size:	200 to 400 square feet
Ceiling height:	8 to 10 feet

INTERIOR SURFACES

Floor:	Easily maintained and cleaned
	Resilient tile
	Sheet vinyl
	Paving brick
	Terrazzo
	Carpet
Walls:	Easily maintained and cleaned
	Vinyl wall covering
	Gypsum wallboard
	Masonry

Ceiling:	Acoustical treatment recommended
	Acoustical tile
	Gypsum wallboard

MOVABLE EQUIPMENT AND FURNITURE

Coffee tables
End tables
Table lamps
Floor lamps
Lounge seats
Plants
Artwork
Wastebasket
Clock

BUILT-IN EQUIPMENT

Information counter or desk
Public telephone
Directional signs
Directory of the facility
Drinking fountain

CLIMATE CONTROL

Temperature:	75°F
Humidity:	30 to 50%
Outside air:	2 air changes per hour
Total air changes:	6 per hour
Pressure relationship:	Equal

LIGHTING

| Quantity: | 30 footcandles/general |
| | 50 footcandles/detail |

Type:	Incandescent
	Mercury vapor
	Special lighting for featured areas or displays

ACOUSTICS

This is a very busy place, acoustical treatment is recommended.

SPECIAL CONSIDERATIONS

A vestibule should be provided for energy conservation and the general comfort of the users. Front doors should have automatic operators. The sliding type automatic door is preferred to the swing type.

AUXILIARY SPACES

Toilets: For visitors and residents.

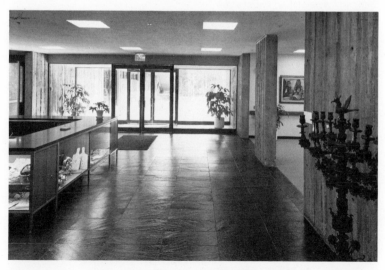

Contemporary lobby and gift shop. (*Riverdale Home for the Aged, Riverdale, N. Y.; Gruzen and Partners, Architects/Planners; Photographer: John Hill*)

Reception Area

In smaller facilities, this space will be combined with the information area, and furthermore a person in the business office would provide this function, as long as there is a view window to observe the front entrance. The receptionist will double as a secretary and will take all incoming calls during normal business hours and spend some time providing visitors with information. In larger facilities, this will function as a waiting room for people seeking entrance to the business office, administrator's office and other departments.

ACTIVITIES

Receiving visitors
Giving out information
Answering telephone

NUMBER OF USERS

3 to 6 people

PRIMARY USERS

Receptionist
Secretary
Visitors

SECONDARY USERS

Office workers
Housekeeping workers
Maintenance workers

RELATIONSHIPS

Necessary to:
    Main entrance
    Administrative area
    Parking lot

Desirable to:
    Social worker's office
    Toilet

Undesirable to:
    Resident areas
    Kitchen
    Laundry

ATMOSPHERE

Warm
Friendly
Relaxed

COLOR SCHEME

Warm colors
Pastel range

SPACE CONFIGURATION

Size: 160 to 220 square feet
Ceiling height: 8 to 9 feet

INTERIOR SURFACES

Floor:
    Resilient
    Easily maintained and cleaned
        Resilient tile
        Sheet vinyl
        Carpet

Walls:
    Easily maintained and cleaned
        Vinyl wall covering
        Gypsum wallboard

Ceiling:
    Acoustical treatment recommended
        Acoustical tile

MOVABLE EQUIPMENT AND FURNITURE

Lockable secretarial desk   Plants
4 to 6 chairs   Clock
Tables   Artwork
Lamps   Wastebasket
Typewriter
Filing cabinets

Telephone or switchboard (there should be some means of preventing unauthorized long distance calls)

Paging system (may be part of the telephone system)

Consideration should be given to the use of portable pagers instead of a public address system to lessen the institutional atmosphere.

CLIMATE CONTROL

Temperature:	75°F
Humidity:	30 to 50%
Outside air:	2 air changes per hour
Total air changes:	6 per hour
Pressure relationship:	Equal

LIGHTING

Quantity:	30 footcandles/general
	70 footcandles/detail
Type:	Fluorescent

ACOUSTICS

This area tends to be noisy, acoustical treatment is recommended.

Administrator's Office
Assistant Administrator's Office

The administrator is the chief executive of the long-term care facility and is fully responsible for the day-to-day operation. This person may have a background in nursing, social work or business administration. In any event this person must be licensed by some agency of the State, usually the health department. The assistant administrator does not have to be licensed.

ACTIVITIES

Interviewing potential employees, residents, residents' families, social workers or others acting in behalf of a resident or potential resident

Purchasing

General management activities

Dealing with local, state and federal authorities

NUMBER OF USERS

Occasionally as many as 5 when the administrator is interviewing a resident and his family. Larger groups should move to the conference room.

PRIMARY USERS

Administrator

Assistant administrator

SECONDARY USERS

Business office staff

Other employees

Salespersons

Governmental officials

Visitors

Social workers

Residents and their families
or other responsible parties

RELATIONSHIPS

Necessary to:	Receptionist
	Secretary
	Bookkeeping staff
	Toilet
Desirable to:	Main entrance
	Offices of department heads
	Conference room
Undesirable to:	Resident areas
	Kitchen
	Laundry

ATMOSPHERE

Cheerful
Quiet
Relaxed

COLOR SCHEME

Pastel colors

SPACE CONFIGURATION

Size:
    Administrator: 180 to 200 square feet
    Assistant administrator: 120 to 150
       square feet

Ceiling height:
    8 to 9 feet

INTERIOR SURFACES

Floor:
    Resilient
    Easily maintained and cleaned
      Resilient tile
      Sheet vinyl
      Carpet

Walls:
    Easily maintained and cleaned
      Vinyl wall covering
      Gypsum wallboard

Ceilings:
    Acoustical treatment recommended
      Acoustical tile

MOVABLE EQUIPMENT AND FURNITURE

Lockable desk with file drawers
3 or 4 chairs
Credenza
Printing calculator
Bookcase
A printout caddy if the facility is using computer services
Wastebasket

BUILT-IN EQUIPMENT

Telephone (with privacy button to prevent eavesdropping by others)
Internal communication system

CLIMATE CONTROL

Temperature:	75°F
Humidity:	30 to 50%
Outside air:	7.5 cubic feet per minute per occupant
Total air changes:	6 per hour
Pressure relationship:	Equal

LIGHTING

Quantity:	30 footcandles/general
	70 footcandles/detail
Type:	Fluorescent

ACOUSTICS

Because of the confidential nature of many of the transactions taking place in these offices, care must be taken to assure acoustical privacy.

SPECIAL CONSIDERATIONS

Closed circuit television has been found useful by some administrators in order to monitor entrances, loading docks, laundry and hazard areas (see section on Security and Safety).

AUXILIARY SPACES

Storage closet: To store confidential material. Closet to be lockable.

Secretary's Office: In larger facilities there will be a private secretary available for the administrator and his assistant.

Business Office

This space will be a busy area. The bookkeeping personnel will be receiving census information daily from the nursing staff; they will be verifying invoices, talking with suppliers, filing a myriad of forms including the important billing forms. The office workers will also be involved in various and sundry other activities besides bookkeeping. The potential for mistakes increases with confusion. Mistakes on Medicaid/Medicare billing forms will result in non-payment. Bookkeeping machines, copiers, typewriters and telephones will raise noise levels occasionally to the point of causing fatigue. The administrator and the department heads are likely to enter and leave the space many times each day. The space must be supervisable, relatively quiet and orderly. File cabinets will be used frequently and must be accessible. Most of the bookkeeping work will be routine and the bookkeepers will remain in their work space most of the day. The secretary, however, will be up and away from her desk often. Residents must be kept out of the business offices; however, a waiting area should be provided where a receptionist can speak with visitors, residents, and staff members.

ACTIVITIES

Bookkeeping
Secretarial work
Active record storage
Collection activities
Paying bills
Answering questions from families of residents
Receiving and sending mail
Updating location board (indicates the bed location of each resident in the facility)
Ordering supplies
General office work

NUMBER OF USERS

The number of users depends on the size of the facility and how much bookkeeping activity is done on premises. Assuming the use of outside data processor, 1 or 2 bookkeepers should be sufficient, one of whom should possess typing skills. Two to 3 bookkeepers will likely be needed if automatic data processing is not employed; 1 secretary will be sufficient.

PRIMARY USERS

Bookkeeping personnel
Secretarial personnel

SECONDARY USERS

Administrator
Assistant administrator
Department heads
Housekeeping workers
Maintenance workers

RELATIONSHIPS

Necessary to:	Reception area
	Administrator's office
	Supply room
Desirable to:	Director of nursing
	Toilets
	Drinking fountain
Undesirable to:	Resident areas
	Kitchen
	Laundry

ATMOSPHERE

Cheerful
Calm
Quiet
Businesslike

COLOR SCHEME

Warm color range

SPACE CONFIGURATION

Size: 100 square feet per worker
Ceiling height: 8 to 9 feet

INTERIOR SURFACES

Floor: Resilient
                   Easily maintained and cleaned
                       Resilient tile
                       Sheet vinyl
                       Carpet

Walls: Easily maintained and cleaned
                       Vinyl wall covering
                       Gypsum wallboard

Ceiling: Acoustical treatment recommended
                       Acoustical tile

MOVABLE EQUIPMENT AND FURNITURE

Desk and chair for each worker
4 to 8 file cabinets (one being fireproof)
Work table
3 or 4 chairs
Mail cubbyholes for administrators and
    department heads (could be built-in)
Typewriters
Calculators
A printing calculator for each bookkeeper
Printout caddies if computers are employed
Postage meter
Scales
Copying machine
Wastebasket
Clock
Bulletin board

BUILT-IN EQUIPMENT

A telephone for each bookkeeper and secretary
Internal communication system

CLIMATE CONTROL

Temperature: 75°F
Humidity: 30 to 50%
Outside air: 7.5 cubic feet per minute
Total air changes: 6 per hour
Pressure relationship: Equal

LIGHTING

Quantity: 30 footcandles/general
                       70 footcandles/detail
Type: Fluorescent

ACOUSTICS

Sound absorptive materials recommended to reduce internal noises and to prevent noise transfer to adjacent areas.

SPECIAL CONSIDERATIONS

Low partitioning is recommended to create some privacy and to discourage idle chatter. A built-in safe may be required if any cash is kept on the premises.

AUXILIARY SPACES

Office manager's office: In larger facilities there might be a need for a separate office manager.

Record storage: The one common complaint from all administrators is the lack of storage. This problem must be very carefully examined. The following is a list of some of the items to be stored:
    Active resident files
    Closed out resident files
    Forms
    Current employee files
    Former employee files
    Correspondence
    Medicaid and Medicare files
    Time cards
Space should be provided for 5 to 8 filing cabinets.

Conference Room

This space is often left out when costs have to be trimmed. Obviously it is a mistake, because generally there is no other place in the facility which allows an undisturbed area for comfortable meetings. A well appointed conference room creates a professional atmosphere.

ACTIVITIES

Interdisciplinary team meeting
Staff development meetings
Staff meetings. Full staff meetings may require a larger space like the staff dining room.
Meetings with regulatory agents
Resident council meetings
Interviewing prospective residents and their families

NUMBER OF USERS

4 to 12 people

PRIMARY USERS

Administrator
Department heads
Residents

SECONDARY USERS

Regulatory agents
Visitors
Prospective residents and their families
Housekeeping workers
Maintenance workers

RELATIONSHIPS

Necessary to:
- Reception area
- Toilets

Desirable to:
- Administrative area
- Lobby

Undesirable to:
- Resident activity areas
- Resident rooms
- Kitchen
- Laundry

ATMOSPHERE

Passive
Quiet
Relaxed
Professional

COLOR SCHEME

Warm, pastel colors

SPACE CONFIGURATION

Size:
- 200 to 300 square feet
  - Minimum width: 12 feet

Ceiling height:
- 8 to 9 feet

INTERIOR SURFACES

Floor:
- Resilient
- Easily maintained and cleaned
  - Resilient tile
  - Sheet vinyl
  - Carpet

Walls:
- Easily maintained and cleaned
  - Vinyl wall covering
  - Gypsum wallboard

Ceiling:
- Acoustical treatment recommended
  - Acoustical tile

MOVABLE EQUIPMENT AND FURNITURE

Conference table and chairs
  to seat 8 to 12 people
Chalk board
Flip chart
Film strip projector
Movie projector
Slide projector
Movie screen
Bulletin board
Wastebasket
Coat rack
Clock

BUILT-IN EQUIPMENT

Some of the listed movable equipment could be built-in
Telephone
Internal communication system

CLIMATE CONTROL

Temperature:	75°F
Humidity:	30 to 50%
Outside air:	15 cubic feet per minute per occupant
Total air changes:	6 per hour
Pressure relationship:	Negative

  Provide exhaust fan to remove smoke.

LIGHTING

Quantity:	30 footcandles/general
	50 footcandles/detail
Type:	Incandescent with dimmer control
	Fluorescent
	dimmer will be useful for audiovisual presentations.

ACOUSTICS

Because of the confidential nature of some of the activities, acoustical privacy must be maintained.

102

AUXILIARY SPACES

Storage closet: Needed for safely storing audio-visual equipment. Door should be lockable.

Office Storage and Supply Room

The supplies typical of all business offices will be stored here. Additionally, there will be storage required for a number of forms unique to long-term care facilities. Inactive files will take up a great deal of space. This space might also contain a copier and the coffee pot.

ACTIVITIES

Storing and retrieving inactive files (personnel records, invoices, cancelled checks, etc.)
Storage of office supplies   Operating office machines

NUMBER OF USERS

1 to 3 people

PRIMARY USERS

Office personnel

SECONDARY USERS

Repairmen	Housekeeping workers
Salesmen	Maintenance workers
Department heads	

RELATIONSHIPS

Necessary to:	Business office
Desirable to:	Other offices (social worker, activity director)
Undesirable to:	Resident areas

COLOR SCHEME

Bright colors

SPACE CONFIGURATION

Size: 180 to 240 square feet
Ceiling height: 8 to 9 feet

INTERIOR SURFACES

Floors: Vinyl asbestos tile
Walls: Gypsum drywall
Ceiling: Acoustical tile

MOVABLE EQUIPMENT AND FURNITURE

Copy machine   Work table
Postal scale   Files
Coffee maker   Wastebasket

BUILT-IN EQUIPMENT

Open adjustable shelving 12 inches deep
Electrical outlets to suit equipment

CLIMATE CONTROL

Temperature: 75°F
Humidity: 30 to 50%
Outside air: 2 air changes per hour
Total air changes: 6 per hour
Pressure relationship: Equal

LIGHTING

Quantity: 30 footcandles
Type: Fluorescent

ACOUSTICS

Adjacent areas should be protected from sound generated by machinery in this space.

ACTIVITY AND RECREATIONAL AREAS

Activity Room

Some people claim that a multi-purpose room is a no-purpose room. In some of the smaller facilities, the dining room doubles as the activity room, however, this is not recommended because the dining schedule severely limits the time available for other activities.

Most long-term care facilities have continuous programs scheduled by the Activity Director. In larger facilities assistants or volunteers will be required to carry out the program. Some homes have a "sheltered workshop" in which residents perform simple tasks for pay, such as stuffing envelopes, packaging, etc. This work is contracted for by outside firms or, in some instances, the work is performed for the home itself. In very large facilities, this work might be performed in specially designated spaces, but in the typical situation, there will be only one room set aside for all activities. Activities will also be provided for bedridden residents by having an activity worker visit these people with the "activity cart." The cart transports items appropriate to the abilities of the bedridden residents.

ACTIVITIES

Musical activities (singing, dancing,
    rhythm bands)
Indoor physical activities
Showing movies
Parties
Arts and crafts
Sheltered workshop
Recreational therapy
Cooking
Card playing
Shooting pool
Board games
Performances by residents
Entertainers from the community
Readings (prose and poetry)
Games (such as bingo)
Religious activities

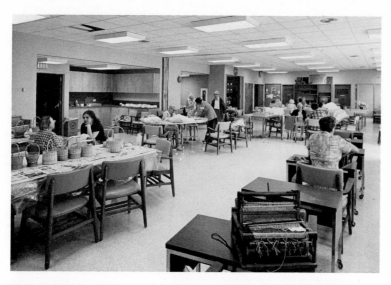

Well equipped activity room, including a kitchen for the use of the residents. (*Daughters of Sarah Nursing Home, Albany, N. Y.; Donald J. Stephens Associates, Architects*)

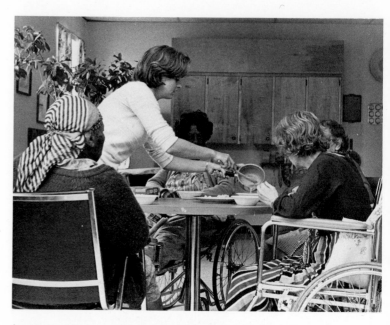

Residents being served food they prepared as part of their activity. (*Photographer: Bobby Thompson*)

NUMBER OF USERS

20 to 60 people

PRIMARY USERS

Residents
Activity workers

SECONDARY USERS

Outside performing groups
Volunteers
Nursing personnel
Housekeeping workers
Maintenance workers

RELATIONSHIPS

Necessary to:
    Activity director's office
    Storage room
    Chair and table storage
    Toilets

Desirable to:
    Resident rooms
    Outdoors
    Greenhouse

Undesirable to:
    Administrative areas
    Lobby
    Hazardous areas

ATMOSPHERE

Active
Stimulating

COLOR SCHEME

Warm color range
Primary accent colors

SPACE CONFIGURATION

Size: 15 to 25 square feet per user
Ceiling height: 9 to 12 feet

Space should be divisible to provide simultaneous use by several groups.

INTERIOR SURFACES

Floor: Resilient
                    Easily maintained and cleaned
                    Moisture proof
                    Non-slip
                        Resilient tile
                        Sheet vinyl
                        Terrazzo tile

Walls: Easily maintained and cleaned
                        Vinyl wall covering
                        Gypsum wallboard
                        (Note: Provide areas to display
                            residents' artwork.)

Ceiling: Acoustical treatment recommended
                        Acoustical tile
                        Gypsum wallboard

MOVABLE EQUIPMENT AND FURNITURE

Chairs
Tables (suited for wheelchair users)

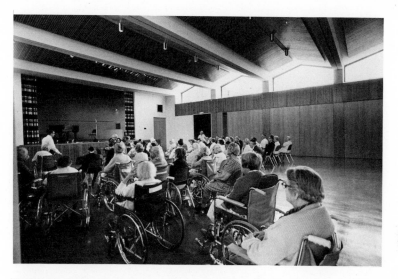

Residents are getting ready to listen to a performance. Note the number of wheelchair-bound residents. (**Menorah Park Jewish Home for the Aged, Beachwood, Ohio; Gruzen and Partners, Architects/Planners; Photographer: David Hirsch**)

Audio visual equipment
Chalk board
Flip chart
Piano
Potters wheel
Ceramic kiln
Activity cart (to provide activity
    for bedridden residents)
Pool table
Wastebaskets
Reality orientation board
Movable acoustically treated dividers
Easels
Rug loom
Woodworking machines (some with
    therapeutic cycle power)
Sewing machines
Clock
Record player

Stage (built-in or portable)
Open storage (shelves)
Closed storage (cabinets), some lockable
Bulletin board
Kitchen equipment (similar to a small·residential
  kitchen but accessible to the handicapped)
Sound system
Service sink
Movie screen (ceiling mounted, motor operated)

CLIMATE CONTROL

Temperature:	75°-80°F
Humidity:	30-50%
Outside air:	4 air changes per hour
Total air changes:	6 per hour
Provide exhaust fan	
for kitchenette unit	

LIGHTING

Quantity:	50 footcandles/general
	80 footcandles/detail
Type:	Fluorescent
	Separate stage type lighting
	if performances are contemplated
	Spotlights at exhibit areas
	Natural light recommended

ACOUSTICS

Acoustical treatment recommended, adjacent areas should be protected from sound generated in this space.

SPECIAL CONSIDERATIONS

Adequate circulation space should be provided for wheelchair users. Use movable acoustical partitions to subdivide large rooms into more intimate areas for simultaneous use by several groups.

The designer must also consider how the room will be made dark for the showing of movies or slides.

AUXILIARY SPACES

Storage Room: For storing the following:

> movable equipment
> residents' unfinished work

  Note: This room should be lockable.

Game Room: Old people like to play various games, separate room would provide some privacy.

Woodworking Shop: Some men like to work with their hands. Simple tools or machines and a workbench should be provided. One wall should have some glass for easy supervision by activity workers.

Activity Director's Office

ACTIVITIES

Planning of programs
Interviewing residents
Observing residents
Record keeping
Ordering supplies

NUMBER OF USERS

1 to 4 people

PRIMARY USERS

Activity director
Activity workers

SECONDARY USERS

Residents	Housekeeping workers
Volunteers	Maintenance workers

Necessary to: Activity room
                    Storage room

Desirable to: Toilet
                   Kitchen

SPACE CONFIGURATION

Size: 120 to 150 square feet
Ceiling height: 8 to 9 feet

INTERIOR SURFACES

Floor: Carpet
          Resilient tile
Wall: Gypsum wallboard
Ceilings: Acoustical tile

MOVABLE EQUIPMENT AND FURNITURE

Desk with file drawer   Book shelves
2 or 3 chairs   Wastebasket
Filing cabinets   Clock

BUILT-IN EQUIPMENT

Bulletin board
Chalk board
Telephone
Internal communication system

CLIMATE CONTROL

Temperature: 75°F
Humidity: 30 to 50%
Outside air: 7.5 cubic feet per minute per occupant
Total air changes: 6 per hour
Pressure relationship: Equal

LIGHTING

Quantity: 30 footcandles/general
                70 footcandles/detail
Type: Fluorescent

SPECIAL CONSIDERATION

Viewing windows are helpful for the observation of the residents.

Volunteer Lounge

The volunteers are important components of all long-term care facilities and are necessary to keep the residents busy and provide additional contact with the community. Volunteers can also provide transportation internally and externally:

- Internal Transportation: taking residents for walks, to the dining room, for medical treatment, to the activity or physical therapy room, etc.
- External Transportation: taking residents to physicians' offices, Sunday rides, visiting friends or relatives, shopping, movies, theaters, fairs, sporting events, museums, etc.

In addition, volunteers will usually assist with arts and crafts, letter writing, delivering mail, operating the gift shop, general store and canteen.

Larger facilities will have a paid volunteer coordinator who should have a separate office. In any event, a lounge should be provided where the volunteers can leave their personal belongings and can relax between assignments.

ACTIVITIES

Meetings
Relaxing
Receiving assignments

NUMBER OF USERS

The total number of volunteers should be close to the number of residents; however, at one time no more than a maximum of 5% to 10% of these expected to be present.

PRIMARY USERS

Volunteers
Volunteer coordinator

SECONDARY USERS

Nursing personnel
Administrative staff
Housekeeping workers
Maintenance workers

RELATIONSHIPS

Necessary to:
    Parking
    Lobby
    Toilet

Desirable to:
    Administrative area
    Activity room
    Office of the director of nursing

Undesirable to:
    Service areas

ATMOSPHERE

Passive
Quiet
Residential
Restful

COLOR SCHEME

Cool range
Pastel colors

SPACE CONFIGURATION

Size: 180 to 240 square feet
Ceiling height: 8 to 9 feet

INTERIOR SURFACES

Floor:
    Easily maintained
    Resilient
    Durable
      Carpet

Walls:
    Gypsum wallboard
    Vinyl wallcovering

Ceiling:
    Acoustical tile

MOVABLE EQUIPMENT AND FURNITURE

Lounge chairs   Bulletin board
Low tables   Clock
Personal storage lockers   Wastebasket

BUILT-IN EQUIPMENT

Telephone
Internal communication system

CLIMATE CONTROL

Temperature: 75°F
Humidity: 30 to 50%
Outside air: 15 cubic feet per minute per occupant
Total air changes: 6 per hour
Pressure relationship: Equal

LIGHTING

Quantity: 20 footcandles/general
    50 footcandles/detail
Type: Residential type table lamps
      recommended

Treatment recommended to create a restful atmosphere.

Volunteer coordinator's office: The work of the volunteers may be organized by a paid staff person. A separate office of about 120 square feet in size, or comparable space within the lounge, should be provided with the following equipment:

> Desk
> Filing cabinet
> 3 to 4 chairs
> Telephone
> Bulletin board

All other requirements of this office should be similar to other office spaces in the facility.

Closet: Storage space is required for coats and smocks.

Outdoor Recreation

There seems to be a tendency among long-term care workers to restrict the movement of residents to within the facility. Obviously, this makes supervision easier. Oftentimes the site does not provide the safety which would encourage movement outside. Physical, emotional and psychological benefits can be derived from excursions outside the facility and, therefore, should be encouraged.

The elements which may be required to insure resident safety might include fencing, trees, shelters, seating, gentle grades, handrails and wide sidewalks. Trips outside the building can be encouraged by providing outdoor recreation. Some of the long-term care residents would be able to play cards, checkers or chess. Another popular pastime is simply talking or observing the passing parade. Residents yearn to observe the community at work and at play. The designer might consider adding playground equipment to attract neighborhood children or the residents' grandchildren.

Screened Porch: A screened porch facing a street would provide residents with community contact and diversion in a sheltered, safe environment. Hobbies, games and other activities can be pursued on the porch.

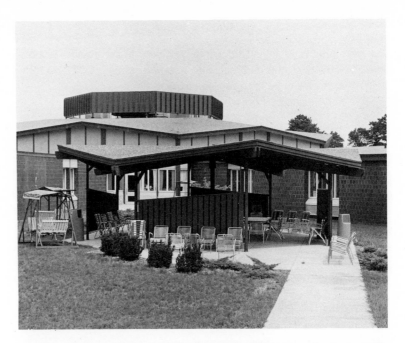

Informal outdoor recreation area with shelter. Wide sidewalks invite walking. (*Daughters of Sarah Nursing Home, Albany, N. Y.; Donald J. Stephens Associates, Architects*)

Swimming Pool: The designer might also consider adding a swimming pool. The major obstacle to this, of course, is how to protect the weak, debilitated or confused resident. It would not be impossible but would require much thoughtful consideration.

Outdoor Shelters: Some facilities wait until the building is in operation and the residents show a preference to sit in certain areas. Then they go ahead and construct shelters over these areas. This seems to be a good idea, since there are many facilities with outdoor areas nicely landscaped and furnished which remain unused.

Security: Security is a very important part of any outdoor development, since some of the residents will be confused and will tend to wander off. Fencing of these areas may be objectionable; consequently, a tightly planted hedge may suffice.

Walks: Walkways equipped with handrail will encourage people to go outside, particularly those who have difficulty walking. Walking will produce a therapeutic side benefit. Walks should have proper

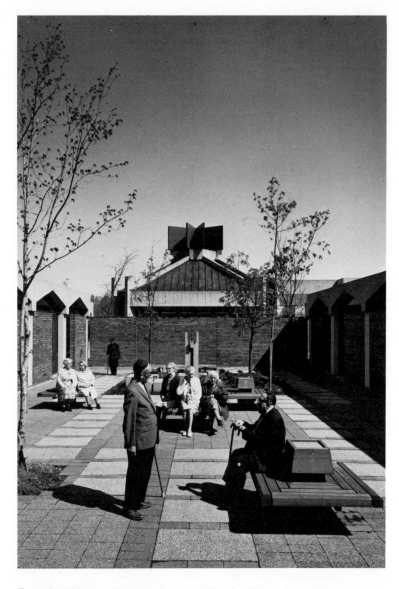

Formal outdoor area with landscaping. Seating arrangement promotes socializing. (*Menorah Park Jewish Home, Beachwood, Ohio; Gruzen and Partners, Architects/Planners*)

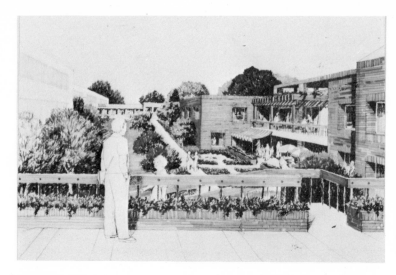

Informal outdoor sitting area providing both shaded and open sitting. (Llanfair Health Care Center, Cincinnati, Ohio; The Hoffman Partnership, Inc., Architects)

lighting to encourage nighttime use and a few benches along the way will also encourage usage. If steps cannot be avoided there should be a ramp next to them. Walks and ramps should have hard, non-slip surfacing. Construction joints should be minimized to prevent tripping.

Greenhouse

A greenhouse as a part of a long-term care facility will provide a meaningful activity for the residents. Not only is the resident engaged in a creative and satisfying activity, but the plants grown by him will enhance the residential qualities of the facility when distributed about the building. Plants also improve the quality of the air.

The designer will want to orient the greenhouse to provide a southern, southeastern or southwestern exposure (in order of preference), and it should be attached to the main building. Certain consideration must be given to those features which are likely to be unique in a greenhouse used by long-term care residents. There are many prefabricated greenhouses on the market in a variety of shapes, sizes and with a great number of options.

Watering   Looking at plants
Potting plants

NUMBER OF USERS

3 to 4 people

PRIMARY USERS

Residents

SECONDARY USERS

Volunteers   Maintenance workers
Activity workers

RELATIONSHIPS

Necessary to: Outdoors
Desirable to: Activity areas
Undesirable to: Hazardous areas

SPACE CONFIGURATION

Area: 12 feet by 20 feet
Ceiling height: Minimum 7 feet with sloping roof

INTERIOR SURFACES

The floor should be concrete with floor drains located beneath the benches. Dirt or clay floors are not desirable, because of the difficulties created by uneven surfaces for wheelchair users, as well as for horticultural reasons. Walls and ceilings are generally of glass.

MOVABLE EQUIPMENT AND FURNITURE

The growing benches should be 42 inches wide, if they are to be worked from both sides or 30 inches wide, if worked from one side only. Some benches should be 18 inches high and some 32 to 36 inches high. The top of growing benches can be of plywood or expanded metal which probably is best. A potting bench situated so that it can be used from all four sides should be about 3 feet square and 32 to 36 inches high. The surface of the potting bench should be of masonite coated with several applications of varnish.

Storage must be provided for flats and a variety of pots ranging in size from 3 inches to 8 inches. Larger pots are available but would likely prove difficult for the elderly to handle. Potting soils or soil components can be stored in bins under the potting table or elsewhere in the greenhouse.

BUILT-IN EQUIPMENT

Sink with spray hose attachment

CLIMATE CONTROL

Automatic ventilation and exterior shading device recommended. Heating will be necessary to prevent freezing in the winter.

LIGHTING

Quantity: 70 to 100 footcandles
Type: Fluorescent or ''grow-lights''

SPECIAL AREAS

Under this heading, several special areas will be discussed. Some of the areas, the beauty shop/barber shop, the gift shop, etc. fill a vital need in respect to the socio-psychological needs of the residents. Those activities which are normal and usual outside the institution should be maintained whenever possible for the normalizing effects on the resident.

Some of the spaces in this chapter could be grouped along with other rooms and located in a central location to create ''downtown.'' Downtown would be a focal point for the residents; the activities taking place in this area would be stimulating and normalizing. Downtown could be developed with very little (if any!) additional expenditure of capital. Corridors could be treated in such a way as to take on the appearance of streets and rooms such as the general store could be given typical storefront treatment even to the point of using "exterior" materials like brick.

Beauty/Barber Shop

Good grooming is essential to a resident's sense of well-being. A shampoo and a set go a long way toward lifting spirits. In this respect, we are all the same. When we do not look our best, our self-image suffers. We may tend to withdraw, to have a bad effect on others; we may become depressed. The beauty/barber shop becomes a socializing space, as well as a center for raising self-esteem. In most facilities the beauty and the barber shop will occupy the same place. Men usually shave in their own rooms or toilets.

ACTIVITIES

Washing hair
Cutting hair
Styling of hair
Socializing

NUMBER OF USERS

2 to 4 people

PRIMARY USERS

Residents
Beautician
Barber

SECONDARY USERS

Aids
Volunteers
Housekeeping workers
Maintenance workers

RELATIONSHIPS

Necessary to:	Toilets
Desirable to:	Resident areas
Undesirable to:	Hazardous areas

ATMOSPHERE

Active
Cheerful

Stimulating

COLOR SCHEME

Warm color range

Bright colors

SPACE CONFIGURATION

Size:	120 to 150 square feet
Ceiling height:	8 to 9 feet

INTERIOR SURFACES

Floor:
Easily maintained and cleaned
Moisture proof
Resilient
Non-slip
Resilient tile
Sheet vinyl

Walls:
Washable within reach
Vinyl wall covering
Gypsum wallboard

Ceiling:
Acoustical treatment recommended
Acoustical tile
Gypsum wallboard

MOVABLE EQUIPMENT AND FURNITURE

Chairs
Hair dryers
Mirrors
Magazine rack

Cigarette urn
Clock
Plants

BUILT-IN EQUIPMENT

Beauty parlor type cabinetry and chair
Barber chair
Storage cabinets
Lavatory
Utility connections for equipment

CLIMATE CONTROL

Temperature:	75° to 80°F
Humidity:	30 to 50%
Outside air:	4 air changes per hour
Total air changes:	6 per hour
Pressure relationship:	Negative

LIGHTING

Quantity:	50 footcandles
Type:	Fluorescent

ACOUSTICS

Noise reduction treatment recommended

General Store/Gift Shop

The general store really serves several purposes, not the least of which is that it provides an opportunity for the resident to once again make choices. The routine of a facility dictates when and what the resident will eat, when he will go to sleep and wake up. Oftentimes an aide will even decide for him what he will wear. Robbed of these opportunities to make the usual decisions required by the activities of daily living, the resident will become increasingly dependent. The general store should provide useful articles, and, if possible, it should look like a store. The resident should be encouraged to make his own choices and should pay for whatever he buys. Paying is important, not to create profits, but to help the resident feel a sense of worth. Some of the more able residents can create "arts and crafts" items that are salable to visitors or other residents. The store might also carry commercial gift items so that visitors can buy them as gifts. The sale of magazines and newspapers should be encouraged to keep the residents up to date. The general store need not be open for business all day and can be managed by volunteers and/or residents.

ACTIVITIES

Displaying and selling of merchandise
Socializing

NUMBER OF USERS

1 to 4 people

PRIMARY USERS

Residents
Salespersons
Volunteers

SECONDARY USERS

Visitors
Housekeeping workers
Maintenance workers

RELATIONSHIPS

Necessary to:	Toilet
Desirable to:	Lobby
Undesirable to:	Hazardous areas

ATMOSPHERE

Should resemble a typical commercial establishment

INTERIOR SURFACES

Floor: Resilient tile

Walls: Gypsum wallboard
                    Masonry

Ceiling: Acoustical tile
                    Gypsum wallboard

MOVABLE EQUIPMENT AND FURNITURE

Clothes racks
Display cases
Revolving and other racks
Clock
Wall calendar
Cash register

BUILT-IN EQUIPMENT

Adjustable shelving
Mirrors
Counters
Telephone

CLIMATE CONTROL

Temperature: 75°F
Humidity: 30 to 50%
Outside air: 7.5 cubic feet per minute per occupant
Total air changes: 6 per hour
Pressure relationship: Equal

LIGHTING

Quantity: 30 footcandles/general
                    70 footcandles/detail
Type: Fluorescent and spot or track lights to
                    highlight certain areas

SPECIAL CONSIDERATION

As in other areas in the facility, the resident user may be wheelchair-bound. The designer must keep this in mind when specifying counters, showcases, shelving, etc., and also allow aisle space for maneuvering wheelchairs.

AUXILIARY SPACES

Storage room: For the storage of extra merchandise.

Chapel

A multi-denominational chapel is an important space for a variety of reasons; not only does it provide an opportunity for nourishing a resident's spiritual needs, but also an opportunity for socializing. Regular worship is an event to which many residents look foreward.

ACTIVITIES

Religious services
Meditation

NUMBER OF USERS

30 to 50 people

PRIMARY USERS

Residents
Clergymen

SECONDARY USERS

Staff
Volunteers
Housekeeping workers
Maintenance workers

RELATIONSHIPS

Necessary to:	Toilets
Desirable to:	Resident areas
Undesirable to:	Hazardous areas
	Noisy areas

ATMOSPHERE

Restful
Relaxing
Spiritual

COLOR SCHEME

Warm color range in dark colors

INTERIOR SURFACES

Floor:	Easily maintained and cleaned
	Moisture proof
	Resilient
	Non-slip
	Resilient tile
	Sheet vinyl
Walls:	Washable within reach
	Vinyl wall covering
	Gypsum wallboard
Ceiling:	Acoustical treatment recommended
	Acoustical tile
	Gypsum wallboard

MOVABLE EQUIPMENT AND FURNITURE

Religious items
Chairs

BUILT-IN EQUIPMENT

Pews (unless movable chairs are used)

CLIMATE CONTROL

Temperature:	75° to 80°F
Humidity:	30 to 50%
Outside air:	7.5 cubic feet per minute per occupant
Total air changes:	6 per hour
Pressure relationship:	Equal

LIGHTING

Lighting should be designed to reflect the religious spirit and still provide adequate illumination for reading. Dimmers are recommended.

Quantity:	30 footcandles/general
	50 footcandles/detail
Type:	Incandescent

ACOUSTICS

Provide acoustical separations to screen out external noises.

SPECIAL CONSIDERATIONS

If fixed seating is used, provide sufficient room for wheelchair-bound residents.

If a raised platform is provided, a ramp is a must to enable residents to participate in the service.

Room should be easily convertible to the different religious requirements.

AUXILIARY SPACE

Storage room: For religious items and extra chairs.

Library/Listening Room

In many instances the local public library will maintain a reading room and will supply all the books needed, including special editions required for various handicaps:

> Large print books
> Braille books and magazines (including Playboy but without the centerfold)
> "Talking" books and magazines on tapes or records

These items can be checked out and taken to the resident rooms or used in the library. The library can be operated by able residents or volunteers. The library should have a supply of current magazines.

ACTIVITIES

Reading
Listening to tapes/records
Checking out or returning material

NUMBER OF USERS

4 to 6 people

PRIMARY USERS

Residents

SECONDARY USERS

Nursing personnel	Housekeeping workers
Volunteers	Maintenance workers

RELATIONSHIPS

Necessary to:	Toilets
Desirable to:	Resident areas
Undesirable to:	Hazardous areas
	Noisy areas

ATMOSPHERE

Passive
Calm
Relaxed

COLOR SCHEME

Cool color range
Pastel colors

SPACE CONFIGURATION

Size:	100 to 200 square feet
Ceiling height:	8 to 9 feet

INTERIOR SURFACES

Floor:	Easily maintained and cleaned
	Carpet
	Resilient tile
Walls:	Vinyl wall covering
Ceiling:	Acoustical treatment recommended
	Acoustical tile
	Gypsum wallboard

MOVABLE EQUIPMENT AND FURNITURE

Tables	Wall calendar
4 to 6 chairs	Reading aids:
Wastebasket	Magnifying glass
Audio-visual equipment with earphones	High intensity light
Clock	Book rest

BUILT-IN EQUIPMENT

Open shelf storage for books and records
Closed shelf storage
Bulletin board

Temperature:	75° to 80°F
Humidity:	30 to 50%
Outside air:	7.5 cubic feet per minute per occupant
Air changes:	6 per hour
Pressure relationship:	Equal

LIGHTING

Quantity:	30 footcandles/general
	80 footcandles/detail
Type:	Fluorescent
	Incandescent

ACOUSTICS

Provide sound insulation from other spaces
Maintain acoustical privacy

HOUSEKEEPING AND LAUNDRY AREAS

Laundry

During the design stage, the developer must decide whether or not to have an in-house laundry. Experience has shown, for a facility as large as 120 beds, that all the laundry can be done on premises less expensively than by the alternative means. Laundry systems are complicated, and it is recommended that the requirements be discussed with suppliers or manufacturers. It must be remembered that a laundry could be open 24 hours a day, 7 days a week; however, enough capacity should be obtained to make this unnecessary, except in the case of equipment breakdown.

A typical 120-bed intermediate care facility can satisfy its laundry needs with two 35-pound washer/extractors and two 50-pound dryers, and two workers working 8 hours a day 7 days a week. It would be a mistake to provide one larger washer/extractor and one larger dryer, since if either piece of equipment fails, the ability to do any laundry would be lost.

Most states require three sets of linen for each bed in the facility, and this is close to being sufficient. The reasoning behind this is, of course, that one set of linen will be on the bed, one in the linen closet ready for use, and the third set will be in the laundry. Increasing this minimum by 10% will be adequate. The purchase of permanent pressed linen will prove to be a good investment.

There are clean linen carts now available which are made to be loaded with enough linens for a nursing unit and which can be rolled into the Clean Linen Storage room. The cart is returned to the laundry once each day for restocking.

Soiled linens should be removed from the resident's room and placed in an airtight container. This is essential for controlling odor and preventing the spread of infections. Care must be taken in the design stage to create a traffic pattern in the laundry that eliminates any possibility of contamination of clean linens by soiled linens.

Elaborate chemical dosing systems are available from laundry supply companies. The chemicals are adjusted to the conditions of the local water supply and eliminate careless use of the chemicals by the workers. However, a well trained staff can do without it and still turn out a good product.

There are at least two alternatives to the in-house laundry. The commercial launderers can provide good service and eliminate the need to purchase equipment and linens. Laundry costs thereby become predictable for budgeting purposes. The latest innovation is where an outside contractor using the facility's linens and equipment does the laundry on-premises at a fixed rate, usually expressed in terms of cents per pound of laundry. This method carries with it two important features. First, the cost is guaranteed; and second, the facility has the ability to return to doing its own laundering at the expiration of the contract. All sorts of contractual arrangements are possible, including the contractor supplying all the equipment and linens which then become the property of the facility when the contract expires. There is no doubt that all systems have advantages and all can be made to work.

ACTIVITIES

Laundering	Folding
Drying	Storing
Sorting	Mending

NUMBER OF USERS

3 to 5 laundry workers

Laundry workers
Executive housekeeper

SECONDARY USERS

Nurses aides
Housekeeping workers
Maintenance workers

RELATIONSHIPS

Necessary to:	Loading area or service entrance
	Executive housekeeper's office
Desirable to:	Housekeeping and laundry supply storage
	Boiler room
	Toilet
Undesirable to:	Resident areas
	Kitchen

COLOR SCHEME

Cool color range

SPACE CONFIGURATION

Size:	250 to 350 square feet
Ceiling height:	8 to 10 feet

INTERIOR SURFACES

Floor:	Easily maintained and cleaned
	Non-slip
	Sealed concrete with steel trowel finish
	Resilient tile
Walls:	Easily maintained and cleaned
	Masonry
	Gypsum wallboard with epoxy paint

Ceiling:	Acoustical tile
	Gypsum wallboard
	Exposed roof construction

MOVABLE EQUIPMENT AND FURNITURE

Heavy duty washer/extractors
Heavy duty dryers (gas operated considered the
    most economical even if propane gas is used)
Tables (for folding)
Clothes racks
Laundry carts
Linen carts

BUILT-IN EQUIPMENT

Utility connections to equipment
Floor drain
Double sink (for soaking)
Shelving for residents' personal laundry
Open drain trough for washers

CLIMATE CONTROL

Full air conditioning is not necessary, although some cooling is desirable; consider evaporative cooling. Dryers need make-up air and should be vented directly to the exterior.

Outside air:	2 air changes per hour
Total air changes:	10 per hour
Pressure relationship:	Equal

LIGHTING

Quantity:	30 footcandles
Type:	Fluorescent

ACOUSTICS

Adjacent areas should be protected from sound generated in this space.

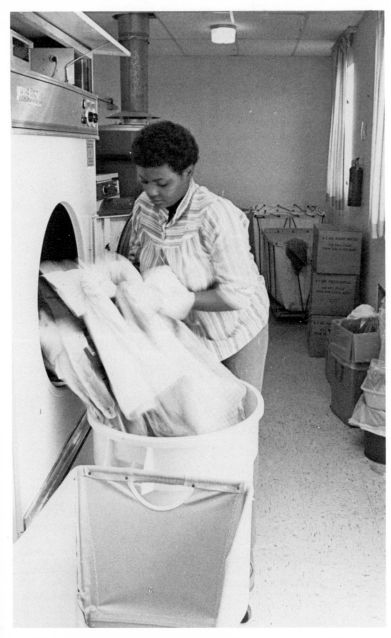

Laundry worker unloading dryer. This laundry services a 125-bed facility.
(*Photographer: Bobby Thompson*)

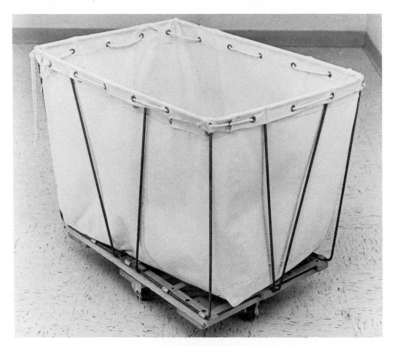

Typical laundry cart used in many facilities. However, this type of cart must not be used for soiled linen because of the odor problem it will create. (*Photographer: Bobby Thompson*)

SPECIAL CONSIDERATIONS

- To reduce vibration, floor slab under machines should be increased from 6 to 8 inches in thickness, or even more; in special cases, consult manufacturer for requirements. Provide vibration isolators in multi-story buildings.
- Dryers should be enclosed with a wall to reduce the amount of heat entering the space and should be vented directly to the outside. This may require a special lint trap to prevent air pollution.
- Some residents prefer to wash their own clothing. An appropriate area for doing hand and machine laundering away from the main laundry should be provided. This area should have some space and equipment for ironing, as well. Washing and ironing provides a social function and an added activity. In addition, it contributes to the residents' feeling of personal freedom and self-worth. This space could be set up just like a commercial laundromat.

119

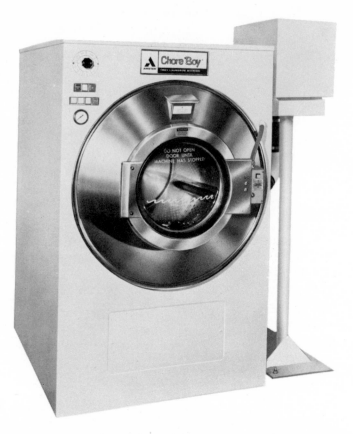

Heavy duty washer-extractor with optional supply injection. Dimensions: 34″ wide, 43-3/4″ deep, 54-1/2″ high. (*Courtesy Ametek, Inc., Troy Laundrite Divison*)

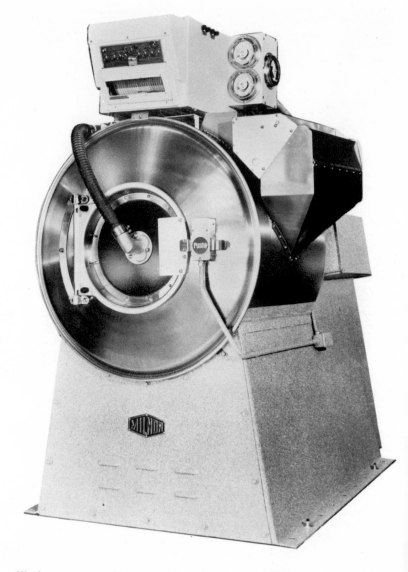

Washer-extractor with center door spray for fast wetdown and built-in load balancing system for high speed operation. (*Courtesy of Pellerin Milnor Corporation*)

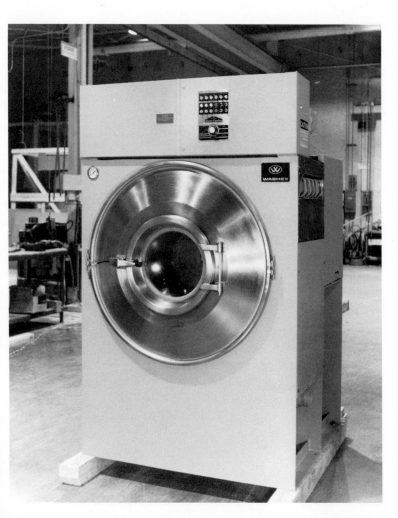

Two speed washer-extractor with auto-cycler to control the various operations. Overall dimensions: 48″ wide, 54″ deep, 78″ high. (*Courtesy Washex Machinery Corporation*)

Soiled linen room: Required by most codes to be a separate room.

Size:	80 to 100 square feet
Climate control:	
Outside air:	Optional
Total air changes:	10 per hour
Pressure relationship:	Negative
	All air exhausted directly to outdoors

Clean linen room: This room is used for the following:

> Storing extra linen
> Folding
> Ironing of residents' personal items
> Mending
> Restocking of clean linen carts

Size:	120 to 160 square feet
Built-in equipment:	Provide about 100 linear feet of adjustable shelving
Climate control:	
Outside air:	2 air changes per hour
Total air changes:	2 per hour
Pressure relationship:	Positive

Storage room or space for residents' personal laundry: The personal clothing of the residents will be cleaned in the main laundry. Some space will be needed to sort out and store these items.

Executive Housekeeper's Office

The executive housekeeper is generally responsible for supervising both the housekeeping and laundry operations. This person should follow new developments in supplies and equipment to meet the objective of cleanliness within the limitations of a budget.

There are "contract" cleaning firms capable of performing all the cleaning required in a long-term care facility. However, many administrators feel a well run in-house operation has many advantages; for one thing, an in-house staff is available for special assignments, and, also, from the standpoint of security, these people would have been screened already.

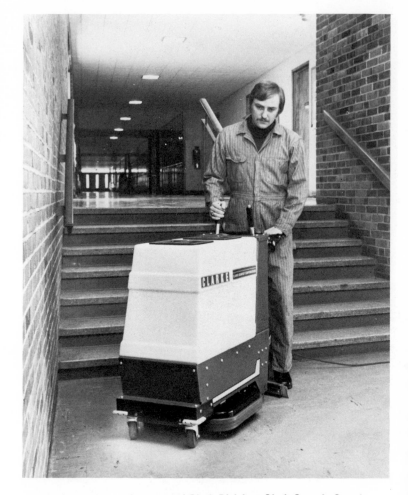

Automatic scrubber. (*Courtesy of Clark Division, Clark-Gravely Corp.*)

ACTIVITIES

Employee consultation
Talking with salespersons
Ordering supplies
Receiving supplies
Keeping inventory
Giving work assignments
Checking on laundry operation
Miscellaneous paperwork

NUMBER OF USERS

2 to 3 people

PRIMARY USER

Executive housekeeper

SECONDARY USERS

Laundry workers
Housekeeping workers
Maintenance workers

122

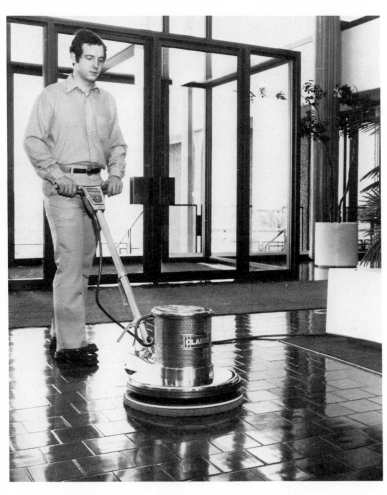

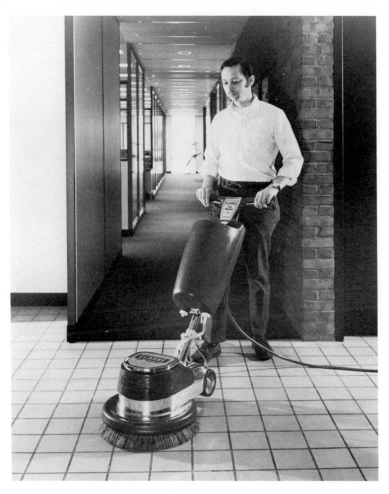

Machine designed for high speed spray buffing and polishing. (*Courtesy of Clark Division, Clark-Gravely Corp.*)

Floor maintainer. (*Courtesy of Clark Division, Clark-Gravely Corp.*)

123

RELATIONSHIPS

Necessary to:	Laundry
	Housekeeping and laundry supply storage
	Cleaning equipment storage
Desirable to:	Loading area or service entrance
	Maintenance department
	Toilet
Undesirable to:	Resident areas

ATMOSPHERE

Businesslike

COLOR SCHEME

Cool color range   Pastel colors

SPACE CONFIGURATION

Size:	100 to 150 square feet
Ceiling height:	8 feet

INTERIOR SURFACES

Floor:	Easily maintained and cleaned
	Resilient tile
	Carpet
Walls:	Any painted surface
Ceiling:	Acoustical tile
	Gypsum wallboard

MOVABLE EQUIPMENT AND FURNITURE

Office desk	Calculator
Filing cabinet	Clock
Lockable storage	Bulletin board
Wastebasket	2 or 3 chairs
Typewriter	

BUILT-IN EQUIPMENT

Telephone   Internal communication system

CLIMATE CONTROL

Temperature:	75°F
Humidity:	30 to 50%
Outside air:	7.5 cubic feet per minute per person
Total air changes:	6 per hour
Pressure relationship:	Equal

LIGHTING

Quantity:	30 footcandles/general
	70 footcandles/detail
Type:	Fluorescent

ACOUSTICS

Acoustical privacy should be maintained. Some transactions may be confidential.

SPECIAL CONSIDERATIONS

Walls should have a large amount of glass for observation of clean and soiled linen areas and the doorways to storage and equipment rooms.

AUXILIARY SPACES

Cleaning equipment storage: Room should be closed at all times. All the cleaning machines and equipment will be stored here:

Buffers	Maid carts
Floor scrubbers	Carpet care machines
Mops, buckets and carts	

Note: provide electrical outlets for battery charging required for some machines

Janitor's closets: Several of these must be located in various areas of the facility. At least one must be provided near the following areas:

Nursing unit	Laundry room
Kitchen	

The janitor's closet must contain shelving for cleaning supplies and a floor receptor-type sink with hot and cold water supply. Floor and walls should be easily maintained.

Housekeeping and Laundry Supply Storage Room

This will be the principal storage area for:

>Cleaning supplies
>Bed linens
>Towels and washcloths
>Hand soap
>Toilet tissue
>Paper towels
>Laundry chemicals

Because of the nature of the items stored here, they must be protected from pilferage.

ACTIVITIES

Inventorying
Ordering
Storing
Dispensing

NUMBER OF USERS

2 to 4 workers

PRIMARY USERS

Executive housekeeper
Laundry workers
Housekeeping workers

SECONDARY USERS

Maintenance workers

RELATIONSHIPS

Necessary to:
>Executive housekeeper's office
>Laundry
>Loading area or service entrance

SPACE CONFIGURATION

Size:	Minimum 300 square feet
Ceiling height:	8 to 10 feet

INTERIOR SURFACES

Floor:	Easily maintained and cleaned
	Moisture proof
	Durable
	Resilient tile
	Sealed concrete
Walls:	Easily maintained and cleaned
	Painted block
	Gypsum wallboard
Ceiling:	Gypsum wallboard (for security reasons)

BUILT-IN EQUIPMENT

Approximately 130 to 150 linear feet of 18-inch deep shelving

CLIMATE CONTROL

Temperature:	75°F
Humidity:	30 to 50%
Outside air:	Optional
Total air changes:	2 per hour
Pressure:	Equal

LIGHTING

Quantity:	10 footcandles
Type:	Fluorescent

SPECIAL CONSIDERATION

The door to this room will be closed at all times and access must be limited to authorized persons only. This must be carefully considered when the keying system is designed. The door must have a closer and a lockset with fixed knob outside and a free operating knob inside.

Staff Locker Room

Safe storage of a worker's personal belongings is a problem dealt with in many different ways. The office workers generally will leave their personal items in their offices. Other workers are likely to carry their personal belongings to their work areas. Workers should be encouraged to use the staff locker rooms, and these rooms will be more widely used if the location is convenient (say near the time clock), and if the area is well traveled and therefore secure. Female workers will outnumber male workers about 10 or 12 to 1, and female workers will have more items to store. For these reasons, the female locker room will be larger than the male locker room. The total number of workers will be about 75% of the bed count for proprietary homes and up to 100% for non-profit homes, but since there are three shifts, it will not be necessary to provide a locker for each worker. Providing lockers for 60% of the total work force should be adequate.

ACTIVITIES

Storing of personal belongings
Personal hygiene
Grooming

NUMBER OF USERS

Approximately 60% of the work force would represent the maximum number of users.

PRIMARY USERS

Workers

RELATIONSHIPS

Necessary to: Employee toilets and showers

Desirable to: Service entrance
                     Time clock

SPACE CONFIGURATION

Size: Female locker room—180 to 220
                       square feet

                     Male locker room—60 to 90 square feet
Ceiling height: 8 to 9 feet

INTERIOR SURFACES

Floor: Resilient
                     Easily maintained and cleaned
                       Resilient tile

Walls: Easily maintained and cleaned
                       Gypsum wallboard
                       Masonry

Ceiling: Acoustical tile
                     Gypsum wallboard

MOVABLE EQUIPMENT AND FURNITURE

Bench
Wastebasket
Clock

BUILT-IN EQUIPMENT

Lockers (suggested size $12'' \times 12'' \times 36''$)

CLIMATE CONTROL

Temperature: 75°F
Humidity: 30 to 50%
Outside air: Optional
Total air changes: 6 per hour
  All air exhausted directly
  to outdoors

LIGHTING

Quantity: 20 footcandles
Type: Fluorescent

ACOUSTICS

Adjacent areas should be protected from sound generated in this space.

SPECIAL CONSIDERATION

In larger facilities the locker rooms may be decentralized and located in various parts or floors of the building. All locker facilities should be barrier-free.

AUXILIARY SPACES

Toilets: For each sex accessible directly from the locker rooms.
Showers: At least 1 for each sex should be provided in or adjacent to the toilet rooms.

Maintenance Shop

A skilled maintenance man is a valuable asset in a long-term care facility. He needs a small shop, more for storage of tools and replacement parts than for actually repairing items, although a small workbench will be useful. Besides allowing space for the workbench and shelving, space should be allocated for storage of a service cart. In some facilities this area may be combined with the mechanical (boiler) room. The maintenance department makes minor repairs, which include plumbing, electrical, painting and carpentry work.

ACTIVITIES

Storing of tools and maintenance items
Repairing

NUMBER OF USERS

1 to 2 people

PRIMARY USERS

Maintenance personnel

RELATIONSHIPS

Desirable to: Service entrance
Mechanical (boiler) room
Toilet
Staff lockers

Undesirable to: Resident areas

SPACE CONFIGURATION

Size: 120 to 200 square feet
Ceiling height: 8 to 10 feet

MOVABLE EQUIPMENT AND FURNITURE

Adjustable steel shelving   Wastebasket
Service cart   Bulletin board
Tools   Clock

BUILT-IN EQUIPMENT

Workbench
Telephone
Internal communication system

CLIMATE CONTROL

Temperature: 65°F
Outside air: Optional
Total air changes: 10 per hour
Pressure relationship: Negative

Quantity:	30 footcandles/general
	50 footcandles/detail
Type:	Fluorescent

SPECIAL CONSIDERATION

Special U.L. approved cabinets are required for paint storage.

General Storage

In addition to all the storage areas already discussed, other areas must be provided for the storage of furniture, residents' personal belongings, oxygen, lawnmowers, gardening tools, etc.

Residents' Clothing: Residents' personal belongings which will be stored outside of their rooms will usually be limited to suitcases, storage lockers and occasionally out of season clothes. Great care must be employed to insure that all items are identified with the owner's name. In addition to the obvious reasons, there is a not so obvious one: many facilities have been found storing personal belongings of deceased residents, because ownership was unclear, and the administrator was afraid of disposing of the items of current residents. The problem can become monumental.

Furniture: Long-term care facility management, which is sensitive to the needs of its residents, will encourage residents to personalize their rooms. This often means that the resident will bring into his room a favorite chair, lamp, dresser or chest which would displace the facility's furniture. Displaced furniture, seasonal articles, extra mattresses, and a myriad of other items will need to be stored.

No attempt will be made to further describe this space, and this is written simply to remind the reader that it is an area to be considered in planning the facility. Most codes require general storage of at least 10 square feet per bed, preferably in one area.

Oxygen: Oxygen comes in metal, refillable cylinders, and, because this gas supports combustion, it should be stored with care. A cylinder of oxygen should be stored inside the building ready for emergency use. The amount of oxygen to be stored is a function of the number and classification of residents, skilled nursing residents being the largest users. Our 120-bed intermediate care facility will have to store four to six cylinders. The reader should refer to the National Fire Protection Association (NFPA) Pamphlet Number 56F for specifics on the safety requirements. To keep fire inspectors happy, it is best to store oxygen outside, in a secure place.

Hazardous Material Storage: The NFPA booklet #101, "Life Safety Code" discusses storage of hazardous materials such as gasoline. The reader must determine first which edition is being enforced before design work is undertaken. The standards for storage of hazardous materials are sufficiently stringent to cause the designer to consider storage in a freestanding building. A practical arrangement of the areas discussed would be a small structure apart from the main building for storage of lawn and garden tools, gasoline, paint and oxygen.

Fire Rating Requirement: Storage rooms over 100 square feet must be enclosed with 2-hour rated walls, ceilings and floors, if these are in the same building occupied by residents.

Refuse and Biological Disposal

Disposal of solid wastes is largely regulated by the local health department. The wastes of long-term care facilities are disposed of by traditional means. Even small facilities find it difficult to do without the large on-premises containers (dumpsters) that are emptied into trucks periodically. Such service is usually offered by independent contractors within a community. these contractors are able to estimate with good accuracy the size of the container and the frequency of pick-ups that will be required. The designer's problem is where to put this container so that it will not be an eyesore but yet be convenient to the staff (especially the dietary and housekeeping departments) and to the disposal service workers. A discussion with the local sanitarian will clear up other questions concerning refuse disposal.

Some states require that long-term care facilities provide a means for biological disposal. By and large this is a useless requirement for it is just about inconceivable that a long-term care facility would ever have to dispose of biological waste—human limbs, organs or other tissues. The only acceptable means of biological disposal in some states is by incineration. Yet some communities within such states have ordinances prohibiting the use of incinerators. The problem may be solved by contracting with a hospital for the disposal of biological wastes. Recently enacted Federal Regulation, Public Law 94-580, could result in new requirements regarding the disposal of solid wastes.

Case Studies

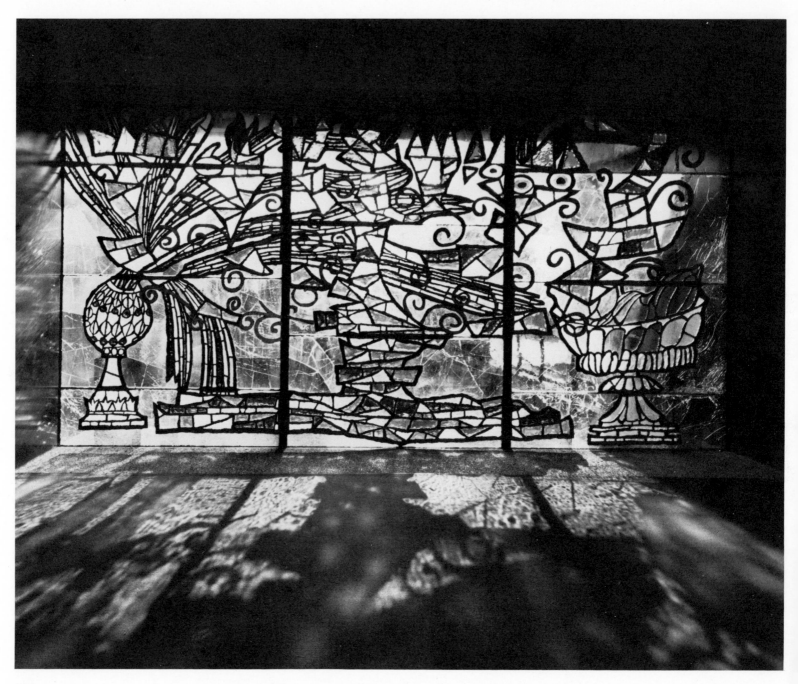

130

5.

Case Studies

OHIO PRESBYTERIAN HOMES
BRECKENRIDGE VILLAGE RETIREMENT COMMUNITY
WILLOUGHBY, OHIO

Breckenridge Village is situated on a 20-acre tract of land donated to Ohio Presbyterian Homes for the purpose of establishing a retirement home and health center. Housing will be provided for the well aged irrespective of their financial abilities in two mid-rise buildings and in five single-story buildings of ranch apartments. There will be a community center and a health care center. The community center will offer a variety of services and programs for the residents of Breckenridge Village and the community at large, including physical fitness programs, a preventive medicine clinic, a home health program, and educational, social and recreational programs.

The health care center, a three-story structure, will contain 50 skilled nursing beds on one floor and on another floor 50 beds for those residents not requiring nursing care, but needing some assistance with the activities of daily living. These two floors place the nursing station in a large multi-use living space called by its developers the "commons." The resident rooms, both private and semi-private, are clustered around the common. This arrangement will eliminate the need of long institutional corridors. The commons will become the hub of activities including dining, recreation and socializing. These two floors will have porches which will overlook the Breckenridge Nature Preserve and will provide residents with an opportunity for outdoor dining or sitting. The porches and skylights will allow natural light to penetrate the interior of the building, creating a warm and residential atmosphere.

The ground floor of the health center will contain administrative offices, meeting rooms, class rooms, medical offices, treatment rooms and an occupational/physical therapy suite. Also to be included is the reception area, a patio, and the mechanical, storage and kitchen spaces. This floor is intended to meet the needs of the entire Breckenridge community.

Project Summary

Architect: The Hoffman Partnership Inc.
Mechanical Engineer: HPI/Engineering
Structural Engineer: Jack D. Gillman & Associates
Landscape Architect: Team Four, Inc.

Consultants: M. Powell Lawton, Ph.D., Director of Behavioral Research, Philadelphia Geriatric Center; Robert Harighurst, Professor of Education and Human Development, University of Chicago

Site: 20 acres

	Approximate Gross Area
1. Housing	
A. 250 apartment units divided between two five-story buildings plus community and related facilities	132,530 square feet
B. 50 single-story, two-bedroom ranch apartments grouped in clusters with indoor garages	66,000 square feet
2. Community center plaza	10,000 square feet
3. 100 bed health care center	55,000 square feet
4. Off-street parking	
A. 81 spaces are provided for the apartment building and community center plaza	

B. 50 indoor garages are provided for the ranch apartment units as well as 23 additional guest parking spaces

5. Landscaped and natural green spaces for resident use, flower and vegetable gardens, fruit orchard, outdoor activity areas and an interconnecting system of pedestrian and bicycle paths

Expected date of completion: Spring 1980

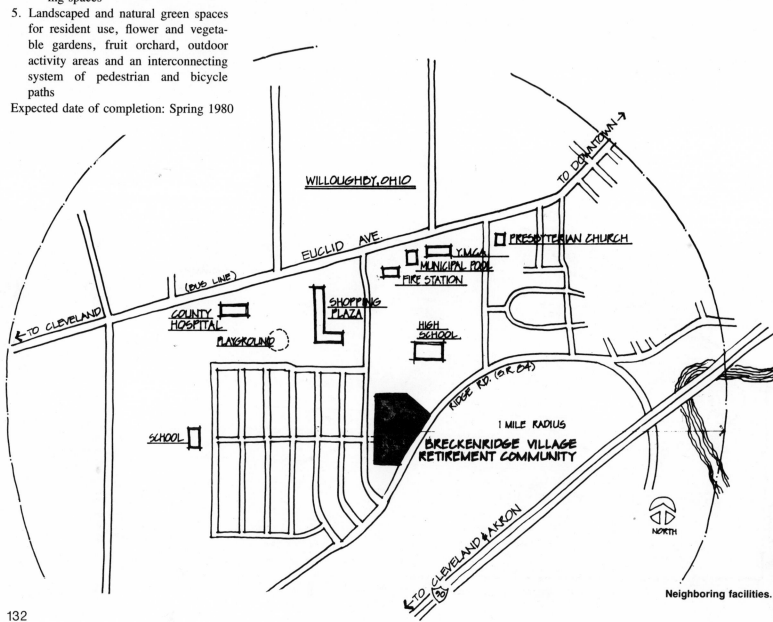

Neighboring facilities.

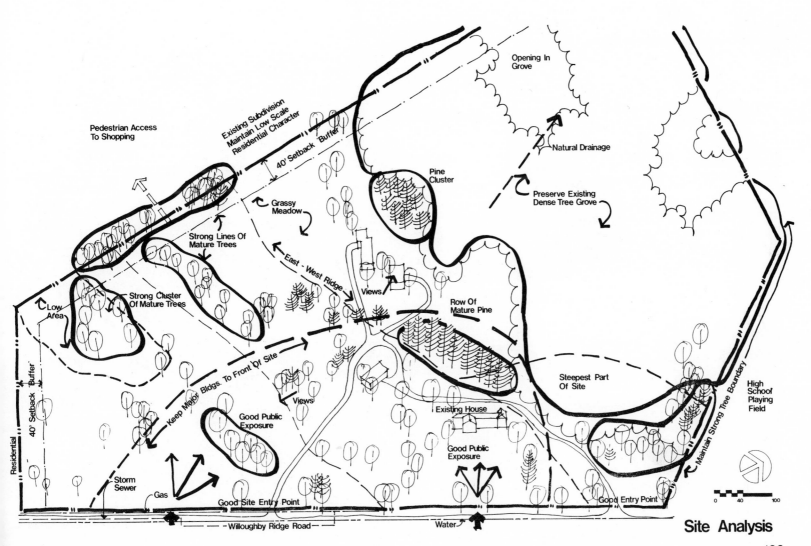

Pedestrian Access
To Shopping

Existing Subdivision
Maintain Low Scale
Residential Character

40' Setback 'Buffer'

Opening In
Grove

Natural Drainage

Pine
Cluster

Preserve Existing
Dense Tree Grove

Grassy
Meadow

Strong Lines Of
Mature Trees

East - West Ridge

Views

Row Of
Mature Pine

Strong Cluster
Of Mature Trees

Low
Area

Keep Major Bldgs. To Front Of Site

40' Setback 'Buffer'

Residential

Steepest Part
Of Site

High
School
Playing
Field

Maintain Strong Tree Boundary

Good Public
Exposure

Views

Existing House

Good Public
Exposure

Storm
Sewer

Gas

Good Site Entry Point

Good Entry Point

0   40   100

Willoughby Ridge Road

Water

Site Analysis

133

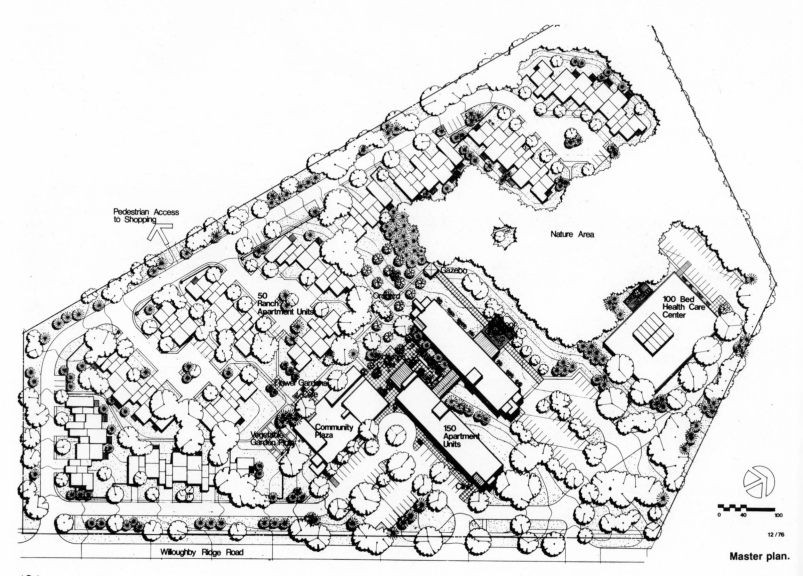

Pedestrian Access
to Shopping

Nature Area

Gazebo

50
Ranch
Apartment Units

Orchard

100 Bed
Health Care
Center

Flower Gardens

Vegetable
Garden Plot

Community
Plaza

150
Apartment
Units

Willoughby Ridge Road

0   40   100

12/76

Master plan.

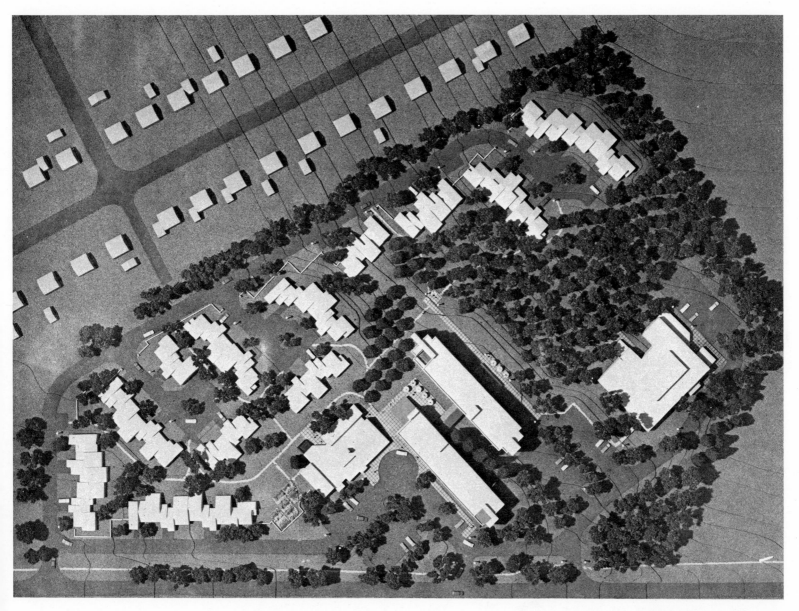

Model photo of master plan.

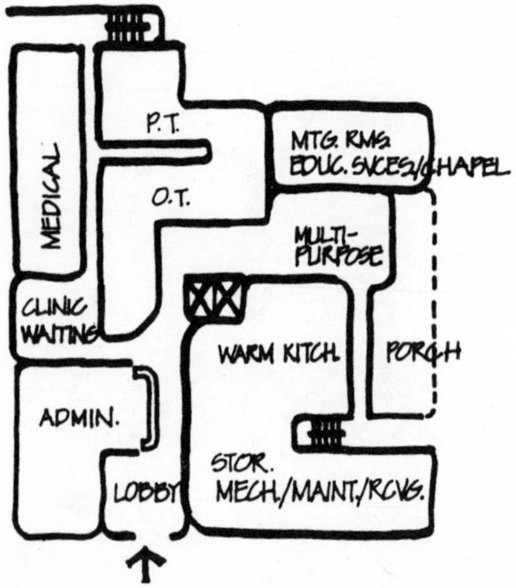
P.T.
MTG. RMS.
EDUC. SVCES/CHAPEL
MEDICAL
O.T.
MULTI-PURPOSE
CLINIC WAITING
WARM KITCH.
PORCH
ADMIN.
STOR.
MECH./MAINT./RCVG.
LOBBY

Ground Level: Clinics/Admin.
1:20

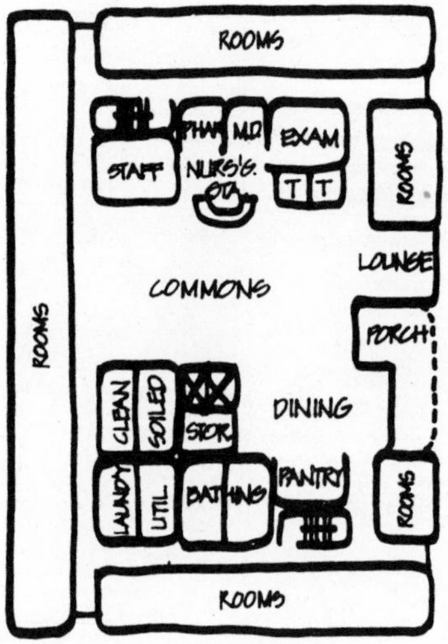
ROOMS
STAFF
PHAR
M.D.
EXAM
NURS'G. STA.
T T
ROOMS
COMMONS
LOUNGE
PORCH
ROOMS
CLEAN
SOILED
STOR.
DINING
LAUNDRY
UTIL.
BATHING
PANTRY
ROOMS
ROOMS

Upper Levels : Nursing Care

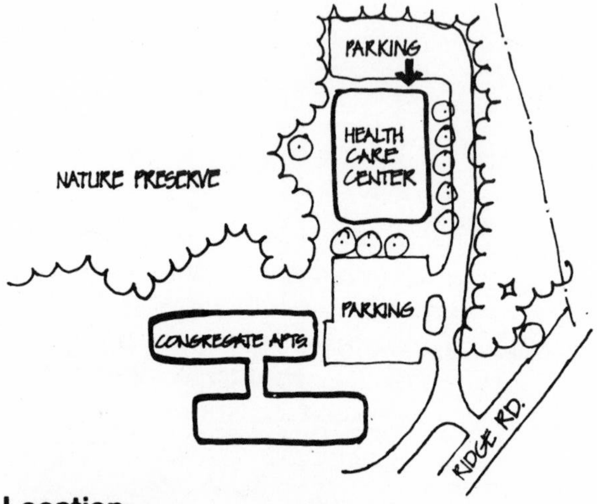
PARKING
HEALTH CARE CENTER
NATURE PRESERVE
PARKING
CONGREGATE APTS.
RIDGE RD.

Location

FUTURE 50 BED ADDITION
PARKING
50 BED SKILLED NURSING
ADMIN/MED. CLINIC/P.T./O.T./EDUC.
PARKING

Concept

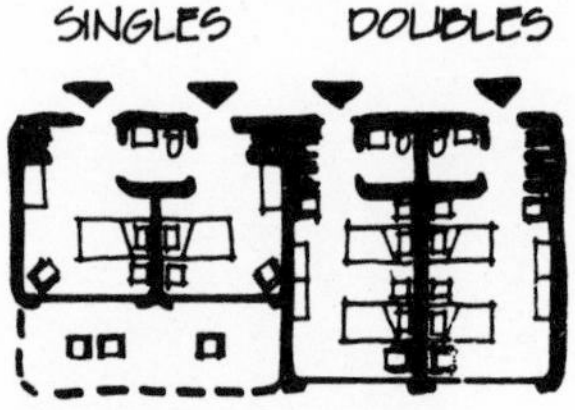
SINGLES
DOUBLES

Patient Rooms
1:10

Health Care Center organizational diagrams.

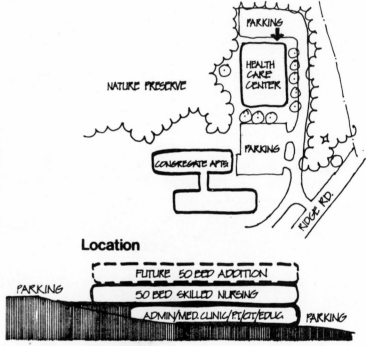

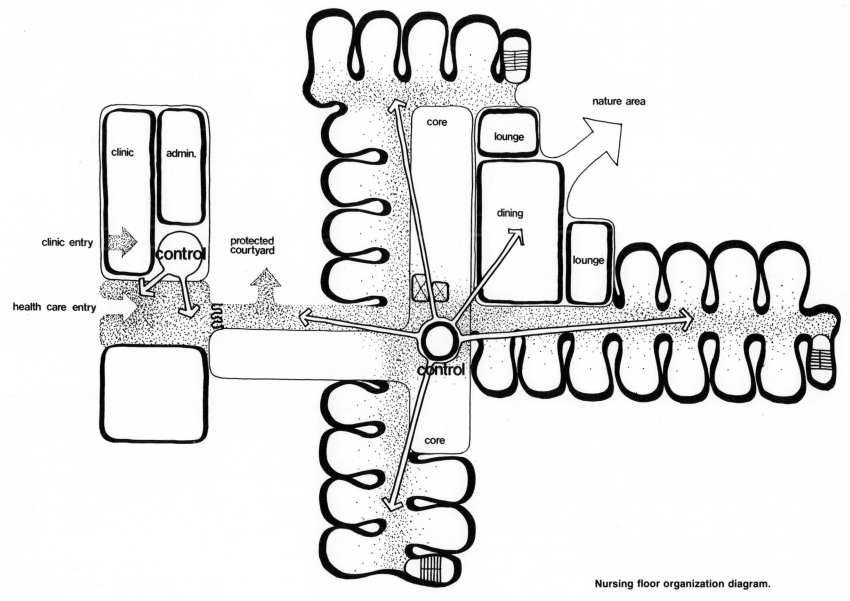

Nursing floor organization diagram.

137

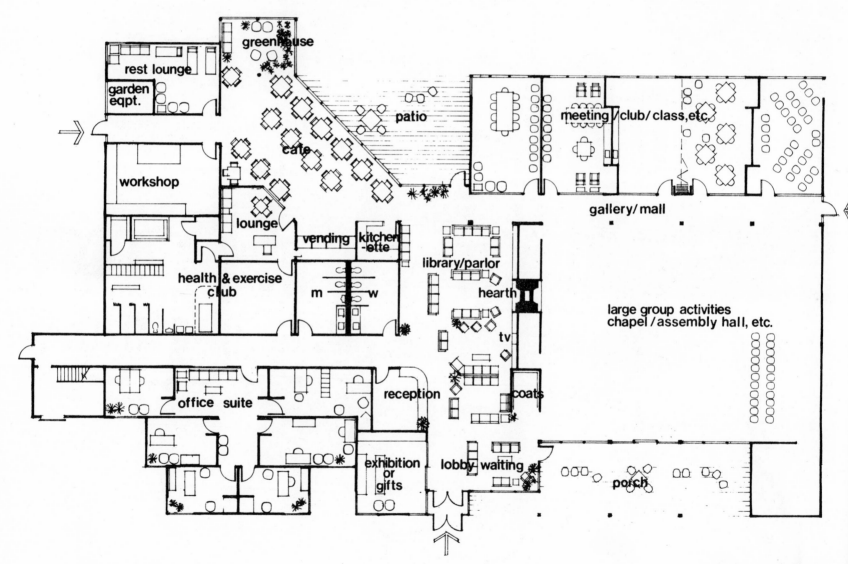

greenhouse

rest lounge

garden eqpt.

workshop

cafe

patio

meeting /club/class,etc.

gallery/mall

lounge

vending

kitchen-ette

library/parlor

hearth

health & exercise club

m   w

tv

large group activities
chapel /assembly hall, etc.

office suite

reception

coats

exhibition or gifts

lobby waiting

porch

Community Plaza floor plan.

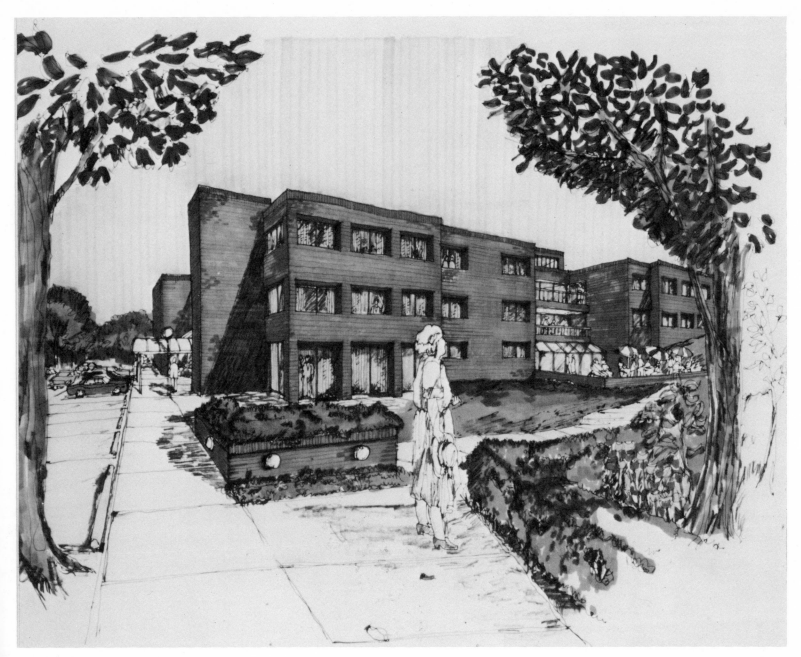

Health Care Center exterior view.

139

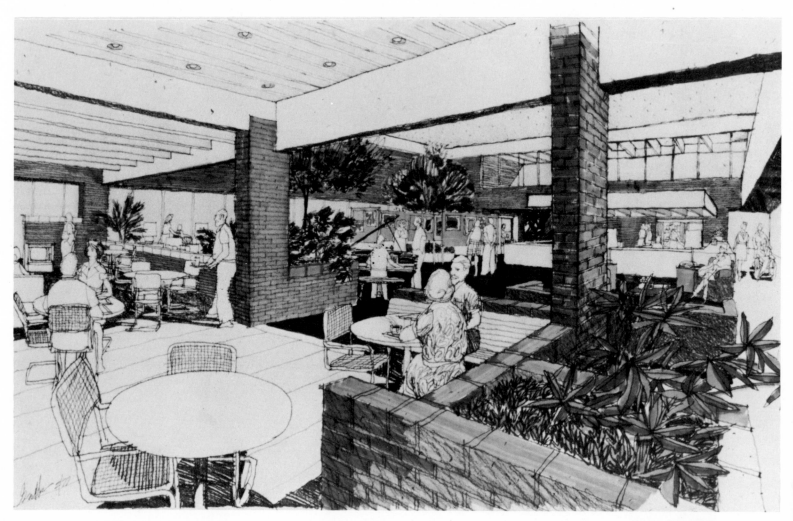

Health Care Center commons.

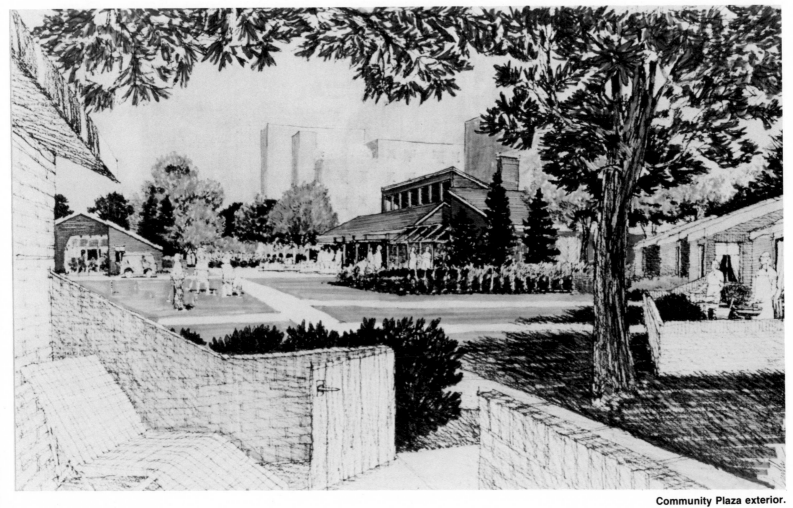

Community Plaza exterior.

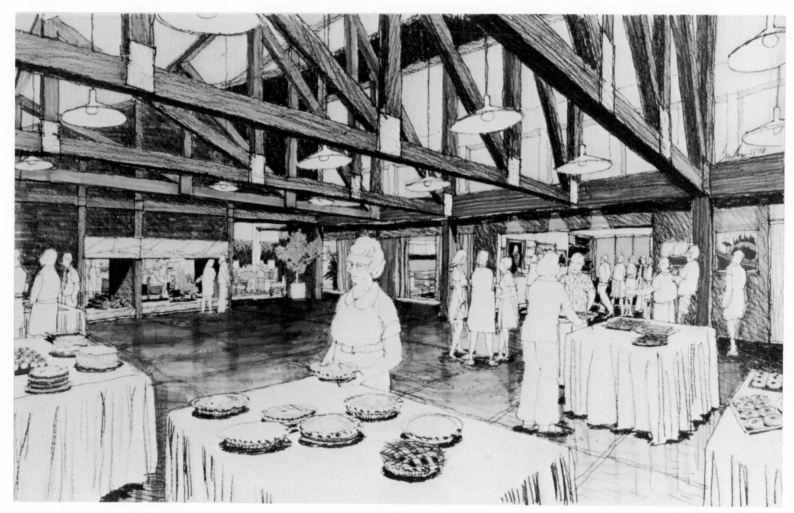

Community Plaza interior.

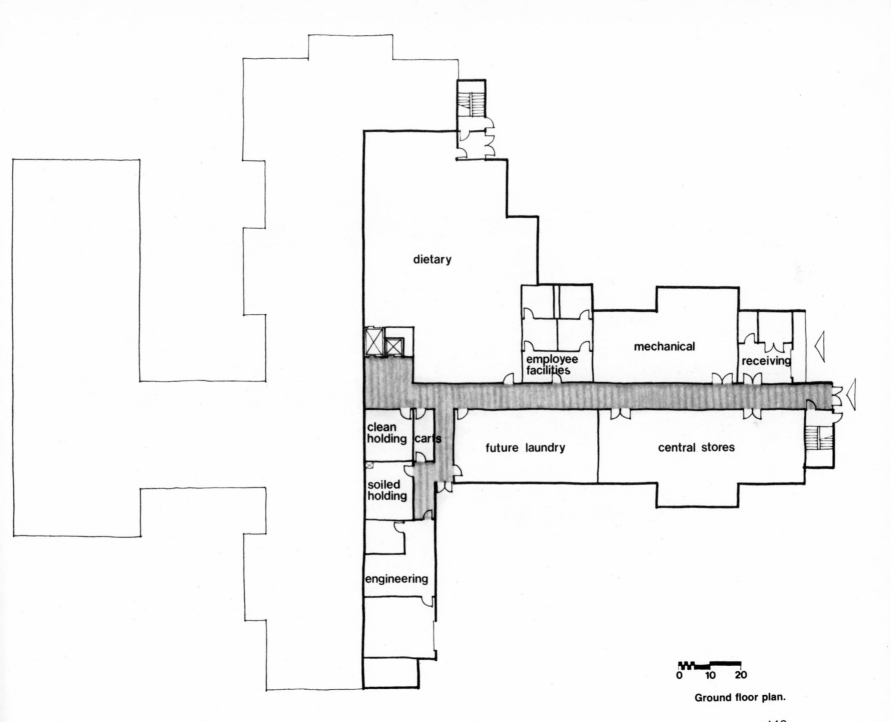

dietary

employee
facilities

mechanical

receiving

clean
holding carts

future laundry

central stores

soiled
holding

engineering

0 10 20

Ground floor plan.

143

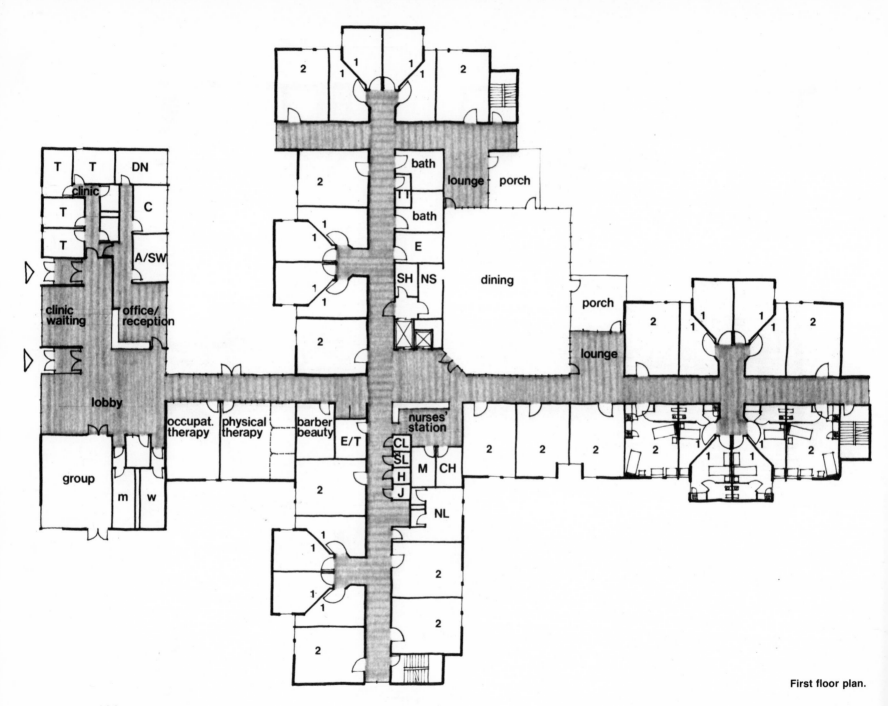

First floor plan.

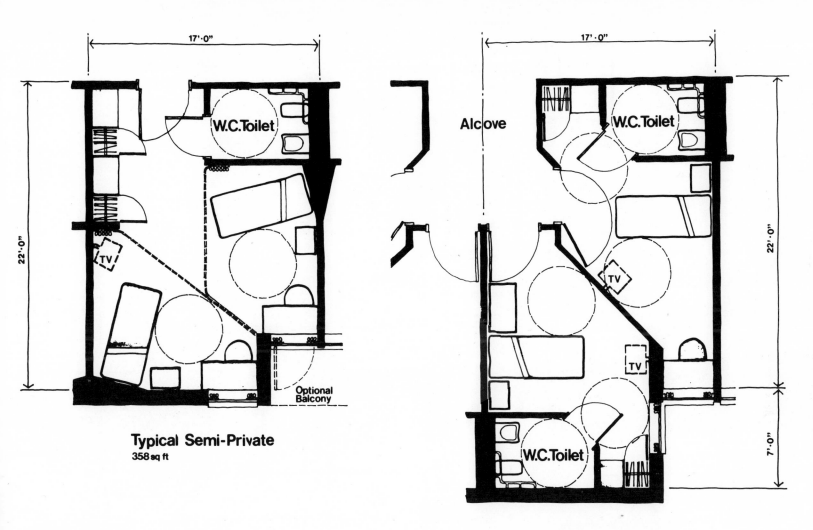

17'·0"

22'·0"

W.C.Toilet

TV

Optional
Balcony

Typical Semi-Private
358 sq ft

Alcove

17'·0"

W.C.Toilet

22'·0"

TV

TV

W.C.Toilet

7'·0"

Typical Private (Pair)
210 sq ft each

0 2 4

Private and semi-private room layouts.

145

MENORAH PARK JEWISH HOME FOR AGED
BEACHWOOD, OHIO

Program and Design

This facility was conceived of as a geriatric center to meet a variety of needs for an aged population in the Cleveland area. Several features set it apart from other long-term care facilities, such as providing a 14-bed acute care unit, a 15-bed psychiatric unit, and a 12-bed, short stay unit, as well as the long-term care unit with 240 beds. Additionally, the facility has its own operating room for minor surgical procedures, a laboratory, a pharmacy, an X-ray unit and areas for providing dental, ear, nose, throat, ophthalmological, podiatry, physical and occupational therapy services. Also incorporated into the structure is a day-care center with its own lounges, dining room and locker room designed to care for as many as 100 day-care visitors a day.

Menorah Park offers "out-reach" services such as "Meals-On-Wheels." The program is uniquely comprehensive in that in the planning process the social, psychological and medical needs of the aged population it serves were given a position of prime importance. The main building takes the form of a series of separate H-shaped pavilions surrounding and linked to a central communal area containing the ancillary facilities. Each pavilion is virtually self-sufficient, in that it contains its own nurses station, medication preparation room, examination room, baths, sun room and dining room with a pantry. In addition, there is a large activity room situated next to the nurses' station (for supervision) and facing an outdoor sculpture garden.

The communal area conveys a feeling of being "downtown." It contains a snack bar, hospitality shop, auditorium, synagogue, a sheltered workshop, library, beauty shop, barber shop, offices, the physical and occupational therapy units, as well as the day-care center. Visiting "downtown" is an important event for Menorah Park residents.

Structure and Mechanical System

The complex consists of single story units with a precast concrete structural system composed of beams and columns with folded plates and double "Tee" members at the roof. The voids left in the concrete frame are filled with brick and glass to complete the enclosure. The interior finishes are generally metal-stud construction with plaster on rock lath, with a vinyl covering in the bedroom units and some other areas. The folded plate gives a non-institutional quality, reflecting the residential character of the area and reinforcing the concept of individual dignity and privacy in the residential units by creating a more personalized space. The building is entirely air-conditioned with fan-coil units in the bedrooms and a central system in all other spaces.

Project Summary

Architect: Gruzen & Partners
Owner: Menorah Park Jewish Home For Aged
Contractor: Turner Construction Company
Structural Engineer: Lev Zetlin Associates, Inc.
Mechanical Engineer: Seelye, Stevenson, Value & Knecht, Inc.
Landscape Architect: M. Paul Friedberg and Associates
Kitchen Consultant: Robert L. Cahn Associates
Interior Design: Bill Bagnall Associates
Artists: Ben Shahn, Glass Mural; Joanna Siegel, Tapestries
Site: 30 acres
Number of beds: 240
Number of floors: 2 (below ground level for services only)
Gross area of building: 189,500 square feet
Building area per bed: 675 square feet
Number of beds per nurses station: 14, 15, 24, and 36

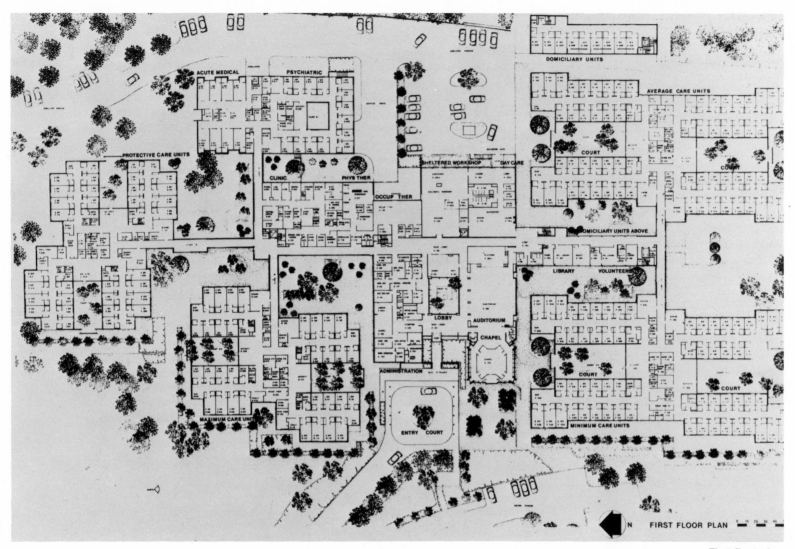

First floor plan.

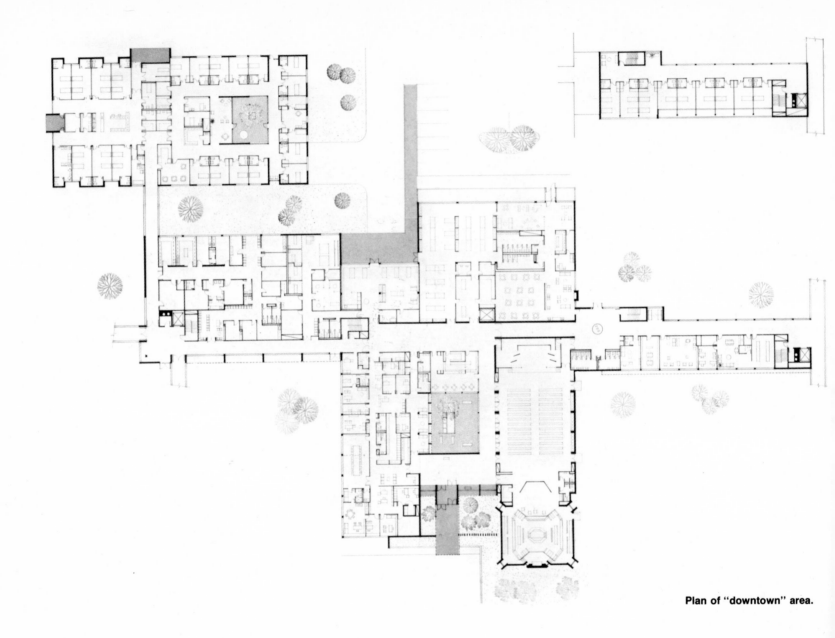

Plan of "downtown" area.

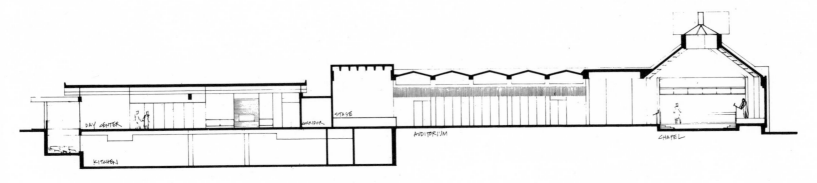

DAY CENTER
KITCHEN
CORRIDOR
STAGE
AUDITORIUM
CHAPEL

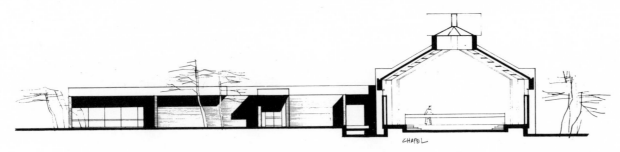

CHAPEL

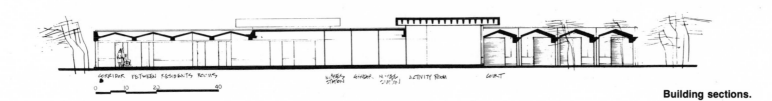

CORRIDOR BETWEEN RESIDENTS ROOMS

0   10   20   40

NURSES STATION   CORRIDOR   NURSES STATION   ACTIVITY ROOM   COURT

Building sections.

149

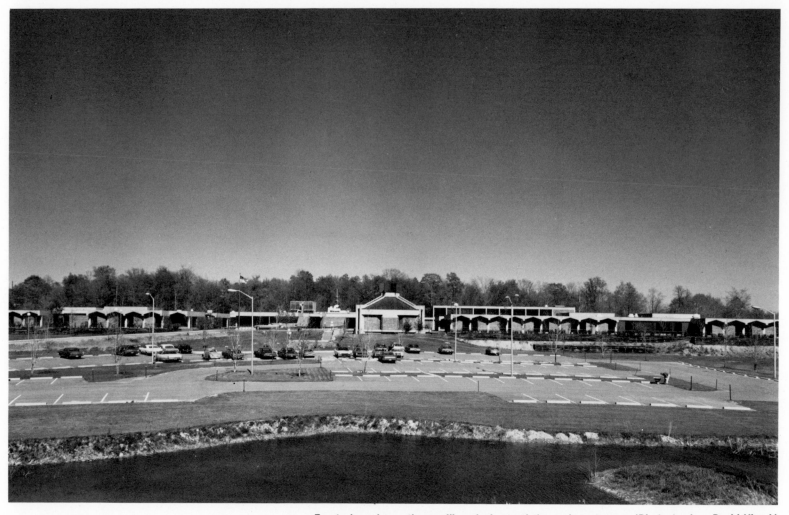

Front view shows the pavilion design and the main entrance. (*Photographer: David Hirsch*)

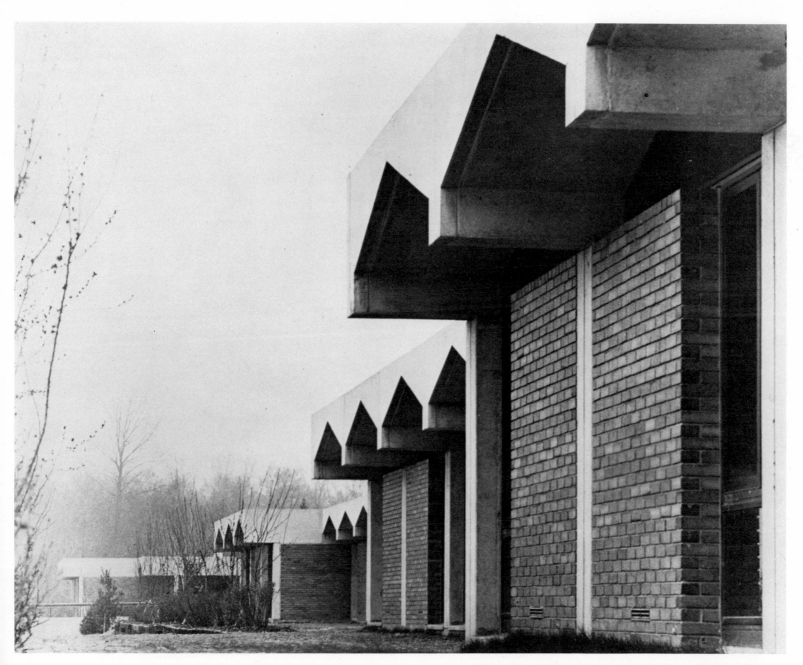

Folded plate concrete roof eliminates need for interior supports.

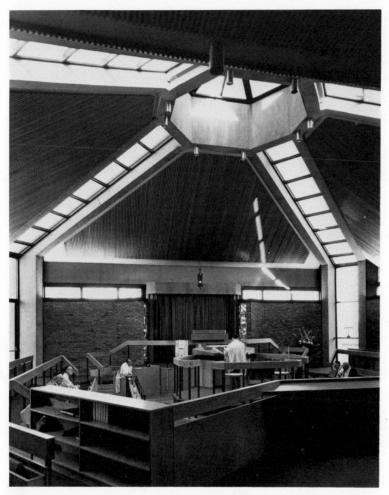

Religious service being conducted in the synagogue. (*Photographer: David Hirsch*)

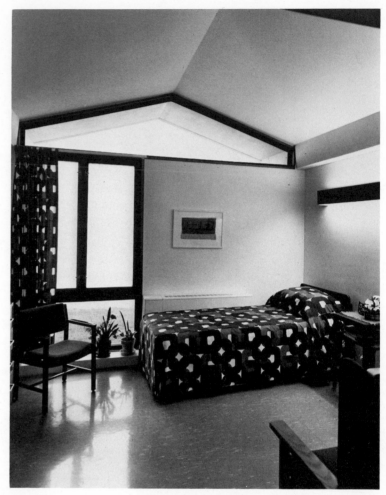

Resident room (*Photographer: David Hirsch*)

152

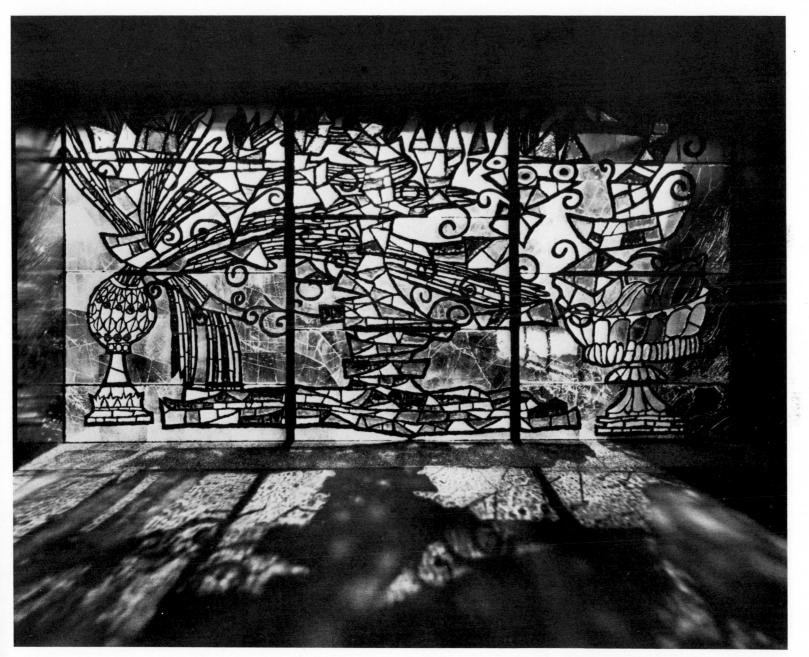

Epoxy glass mural (19′ by 9′) by Ben Shahn

TRIAD UNITED METHODIST HOME
WINSTON-SALEM, NORTH CAROLINA

Design Philosophy and Goals

- Residents should be able to see some of the daily activity of the home from their rooms: people coming and going, the arrival of visitors, recreational activities, etc.
- Walking through the home should be easy and pleasant. There should be a choice of routes, interesting views from corridors, and the opportunity to meet people along the way.
- Full advantage should be taken of the unique character of the site: the slope, the views, and the large trees.
- The cottages and duplexes, while easily accessible by car, should not be isolated from the community activities.
- The home should be able to grow in such a way that it is complete at each stage but can adapt to future needs.

Organization on the Site

One part of the site is particularly well-suited to the achievement of the design goals. The shape of the land near the center of the site creates a natural amphitheatre facing a cluster of magnificent trees. At the bottom of the slope the creek will be dammed to make a small lake, around which the common rooms will be grouped. The pedestrian street will bend around the lake and connect the common rooms. Elevators on the pedestrian streets will serve the corridors of the residential units, which will extend away from the lake into the slope. Each corridor will end at grade level where there will be doors to gardening areas, terraces, and pathways within the courtyards. At the top of the slope, where the height of the residential buildings will be only one story, the cottages and duplexes will complete the enclosure of the courtyards. A road circling the complex will give private car access to cottages and duplexes, as well as providing a highly visible approach to the main entrance. The first phase of project now under construction will consist of 85 residential units and 20 health care beds. The home will grow in stages to the maximum capacity of 400 residents, eventually completely encircling the lake.

Project Summary

Architect: Newman, Calloway, Johnson, Van Etten, Winfree Associates
Planning Consultant: Harvey Johnson
Landscape Architect: McNeely Associates
Number of beds: 20 nursing beds, 85 residential units
Gross area of building: 93,000 square feet
Number of floors: nursing wings: 1 floor; residential living: 4 floors
Parking spaces: 111

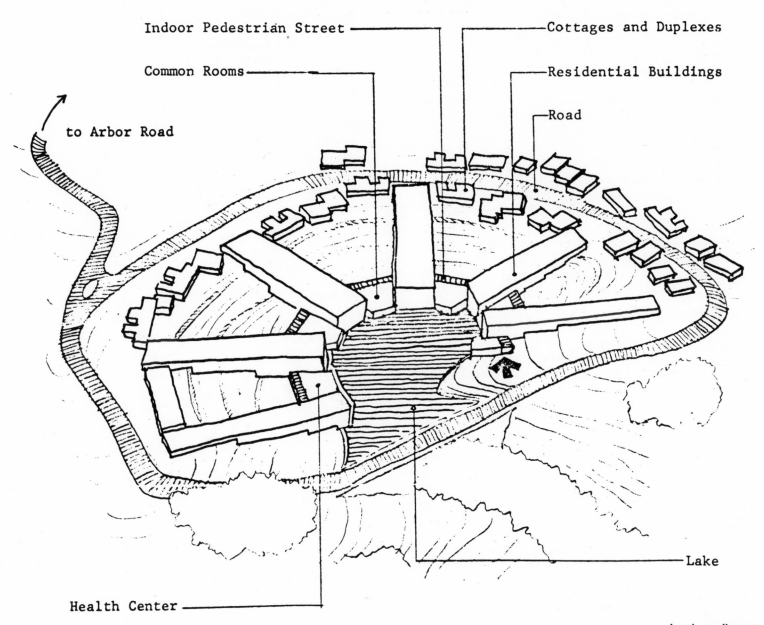

Indoor Pedestrian Street

Common Rooms

to Arbor Road

Cottages and Duplexes

Residential Buildings

Road

Lake

Health Center

Land use diagram.

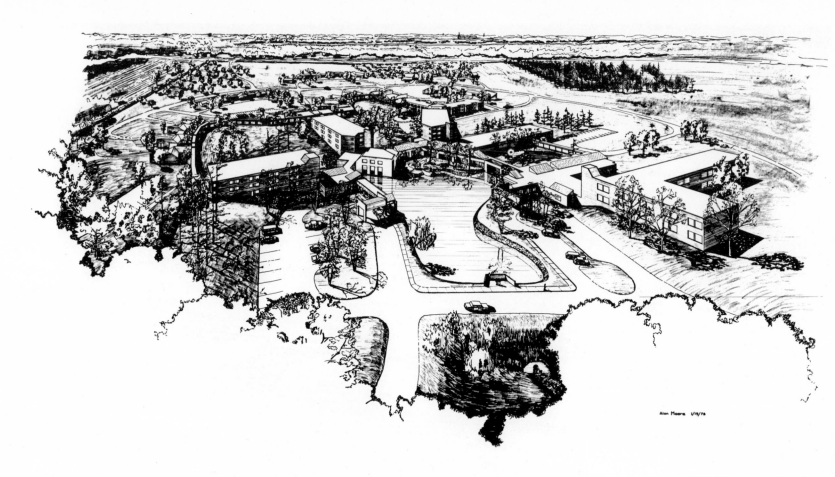

Perspective view of project.

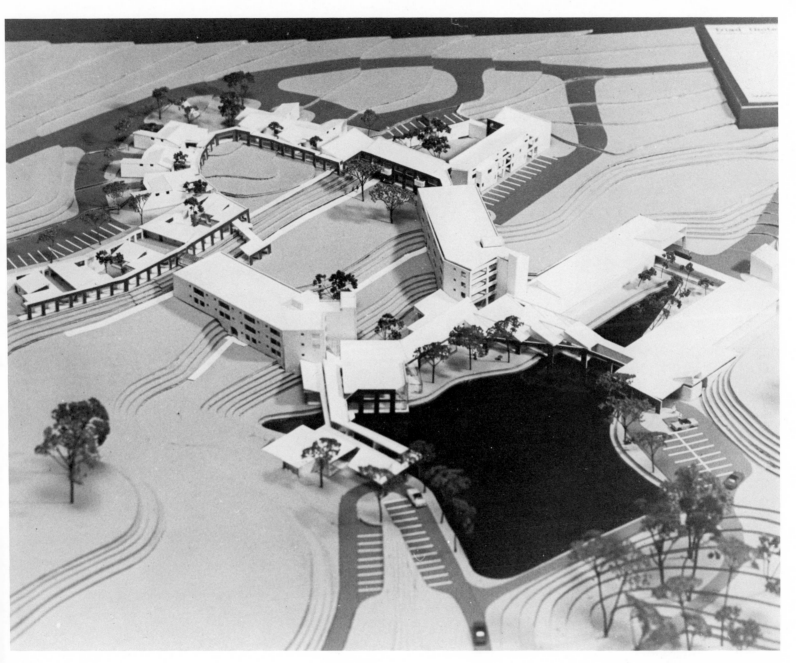

Model photo of project.

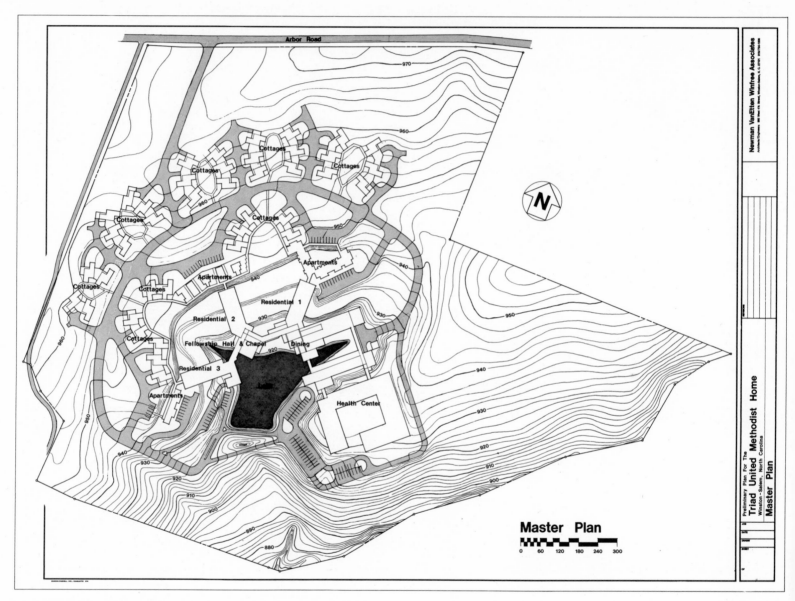

Within the plan, visible labels include:

Arbor Road

Cottages

Apartments

Residential 1
Residential 2
Residential 3

Fellowship Hall & Chapel

Dining

Health Center

Master Plan

0 60 120 180 240 300

Newman VanEtten Winfree Associates

Preliminary Plan For The
Triad United Methodist Home
Winston-Salem, North Carolina
Master Plan

Master plan.

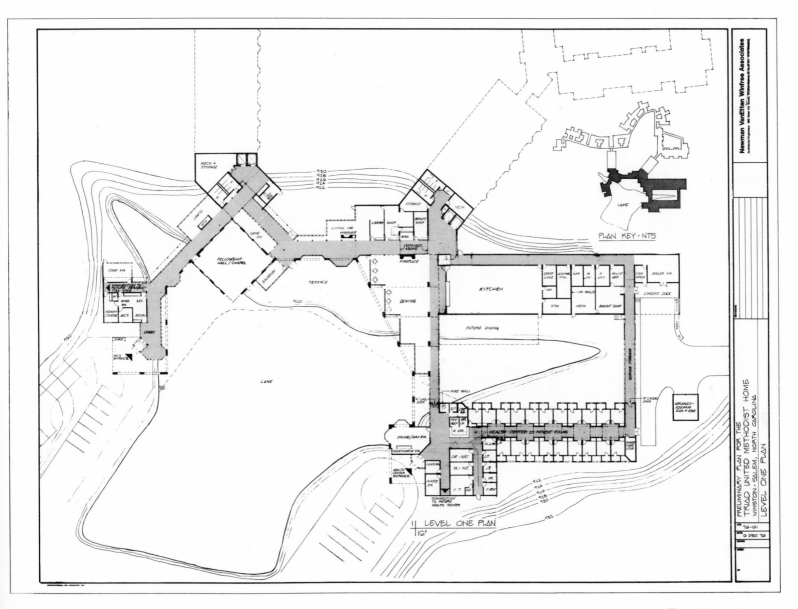

PLAN KEY - NTS

PRELIMINARY PLAN FOR THE
TRIAD UNITED METHODIST HOME
WINSTON-SALEM, NORTH CAROLINA

LEVEL ONE PLAN

MECH +
STORAGE

CONF. RM.

WORK RM.   SEC.

ADMINI-   RECPN.
STRATOR   ACCT.

LOBBY

FELLOWSHIP
HALL / CHAPEL

GAME RM.

SOLARIUM

TERRACE

DINING

LAKE

LIVING RM.
FIREPLACE

HALL

SKYLIGHT
ABOVE

FIREPLACE

LIBRARY   SHOP

BEAUTY
SHOP

STORAGE

MECH.

KITCHEN

STAFF
LNGE.

OFF.

STOR.   MECH.   MAINT SHOP

FUTURE DINING

FIRE WALL

LOADING DOCK

BOILER RM.

SERVICE DRIVE

GROUNDS-
KEEPING
GAR. + STOR.

DINING / DAY RM.

NOURISHMENT STA.

HEALTH
CENTER
ENTRANCE.

HEALTH CENTER 25 PATIENT ROOMS

CONNECTION
TO FUTURE
HEALTH CENTER

LEVEL ONE PLAN
1/16"

Floor plan of first phase.

HEBREW HOME FOR THE AGED AT RIVERDALE
GOLDFINE PAVILLION
BRONX, NEW YORK

Program Requirements

A two-stage building program was planned to provide for new facilities and the renovation of existing facilities, to develop the home into a more livable and efficient unit and transform all resident care, within both old and new buildings, into an arrangement of a maximum of two beds per room, with many single rooms.

Solution

Stage 1 of the program, comprising 80,000 square feet of new construction, provides for the erection of a five-story nursing addition, a one-story connecting wing to the existing home, and the creation of a new terrace garden as the focal point of the new complex. The 140 new beds to be provided by the addition will not, in effect, increase the home's overall bed capacity but rather are aimed at relieving the existing crowded conditions and at the conversion of the old building into the two-beds per room system. However, within the new wing, there will be a total of 60 single bedrooms and 40 two-bed rooms, all with private baths.

The addition is located to the west of the old building and below the crest of the gently sloping site, giving residents a panoramic view of the Hudson River and the Jersey Palisades and also making it possible to keep the roof lines of both structures at the 'same height.

Ancillary Areas

The first and second floors are devoted to new administrative offices, a sheltered workshop, a dining room, an occupational therapy suite, a board room and miscellaneous reception services. Within the addition, a new main entrance to the home was created at the ground level. From the main entrance lobby, the two-story high sheltered workshop area is immediately visible providing a point of interest to visitors.

Nursing Units

Self-contained nursing units, each containing 40 beds, occupy the upper three stories of the addition. Within a compact service-core plan, each floor has its bedrooms to the perimeter of the building. The center or core of the floor contains medical services, treatment rooms, nurses station, dining area, and various storage and utility facilities. Corridor space is reduced to a minimum.

To help provide for a more residential character, while still maintaining the institutional necessities, all interior corridors lead into corner balconies, permitting natural light into the interior of the building and also providing for quick and easy access to the sun and the view. By reversing every other floor, balconies are formed in such a way that a maximum of light and view is achieved.

Connecting Wing

The one-story connecting wing forms an enclosed passageway, above grade, and acts as a service and personnel route between the old and the new buildings. Meeting rooms, sitting areas and a fireplace make this the new focus of the entire home. The roof of the connecting wing was developed into a terrace garden to provide a pleasant sitting and recreational area for patients and visitors. Features of its design include a sunken garden, raised planting boxes surrounding the sitting area, and an outdoor barbecue pit.

Construction/Materials

Construction is poured concrete frame, with board-formed concrete exterior wall surfaces. Infill panels are of solar glass and red brick, matching the brick of the original building. Brick is also used for paving on the terrace and in main entrance lobbies.

Air-Conditioning

This phase of the construction made provisions for air-conditioning the old central dining hall, as well as locating a central chilled water plant for all future air-conditioning in conjunction with updating the central boiler plant.

Project Summary

Architect: Gruzen & Partners
Owner: Hebrew Home for the Aged
Landscape Architect: M. Paul Friedberg and Associates
Structural Engineer: Paul P. Valerio Associates
Mechanical/Electrical Engineer: Seelye, Stevenson,
   Value & Knecht, Inc.

General Contractor: Valridge Construction Co.
Site: 32 acres
Number of beds: 140
Number of floors: 5
Gross area of building: 80,000 square feet
Gross area per bed: 571 square feet

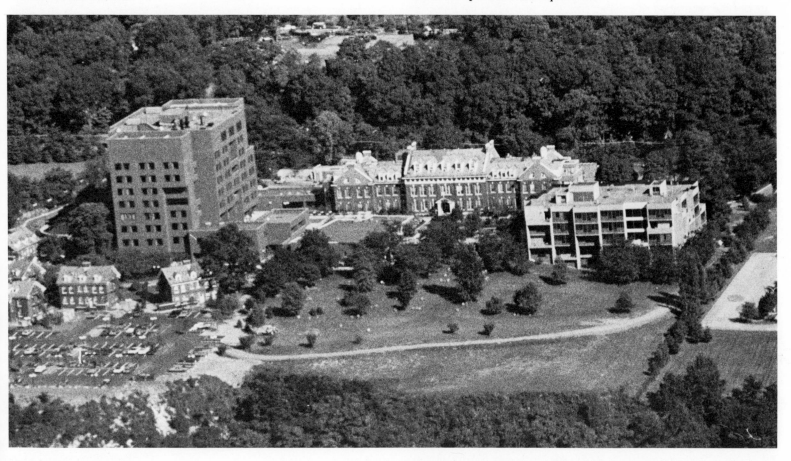

Aerial view of entire complex. On the left side is the newest addition, the Palisades Nursing Home. In the middle is the original turn of the century mansion. The Goldfine Pavilion is located on the extreme right.

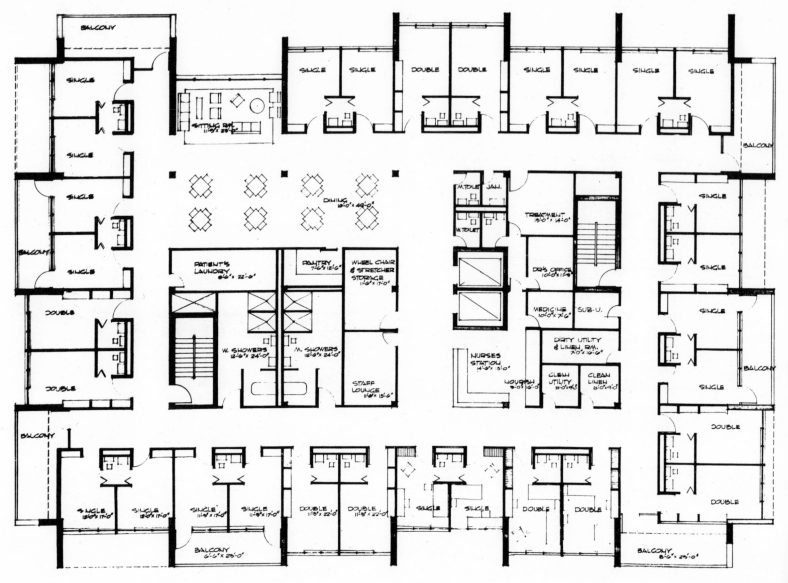

Typical nursing floor.

162

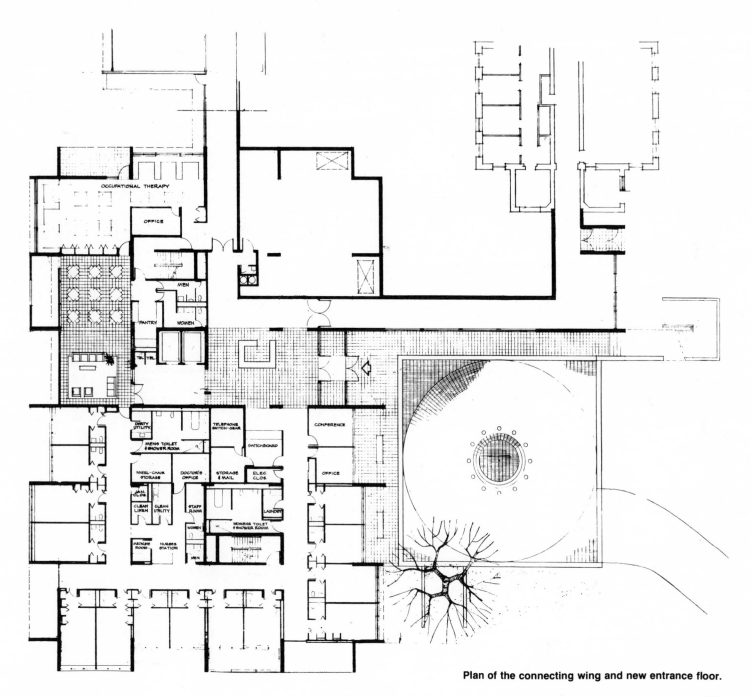

OCCUPATIONAL THERAPY

OFFICE

MEN

PANTRY   WOMEN

TEL. TEL.

DIRTY
UTILITY

TELEPHONE
SWITCH-GEAR

CONFERENCE

MENS TOILET
& SHOWER ROOM

SWITCHBOARD

WHEEL-CHAIR
STORAGE

DOCTOR'S
OFFICE

STORAGE
& MAIL

ELEC.
CLOS.

OFFICE

JAN.
CLOS.

CLEAN
LINEN

CLEAN
UTILITY

STAFF
ROOM

LAUNDRY

WOMENS TOILET
& SHOWER ROOM

WOMEN

MEDICINE
ROOM

NURSES
STATION

MEN

Plan of the connecting wing and new entrance floor.

163

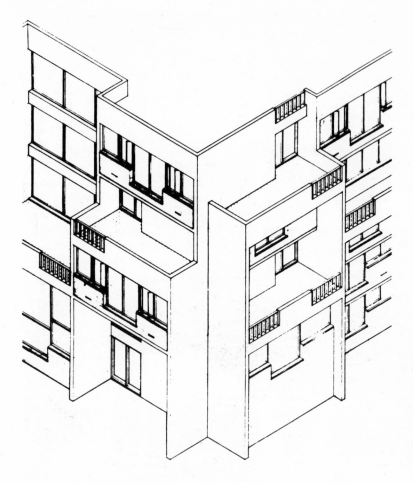

Isometric view of corner showing private and public balconies.

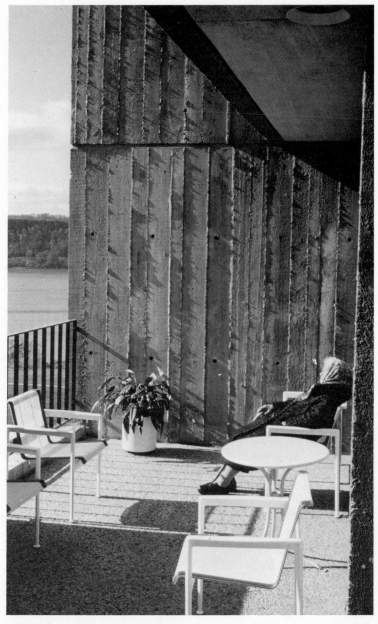

View of one of the balconies overlooking the Hudson River. Note the texture of the concrete walls.

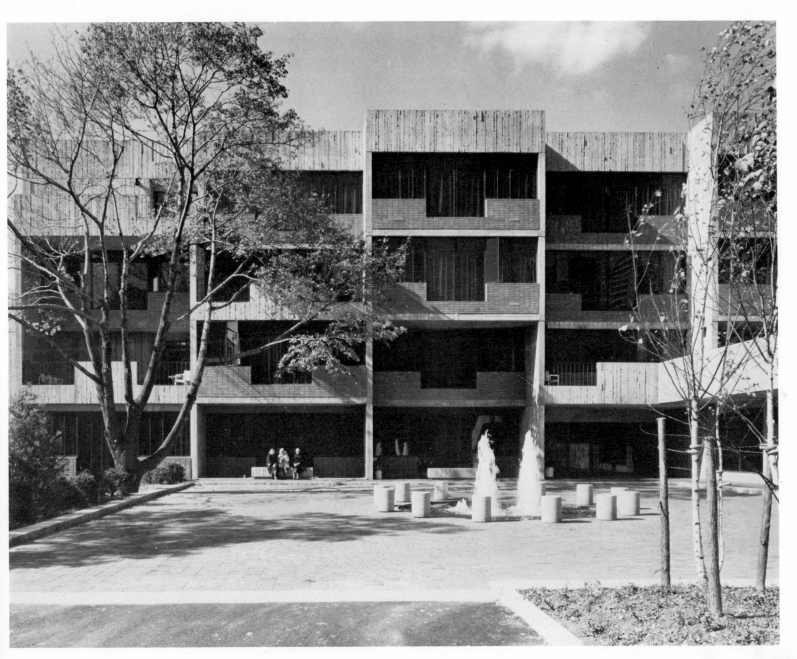

Entrance plaza with fountains and outdoor sitting areas.

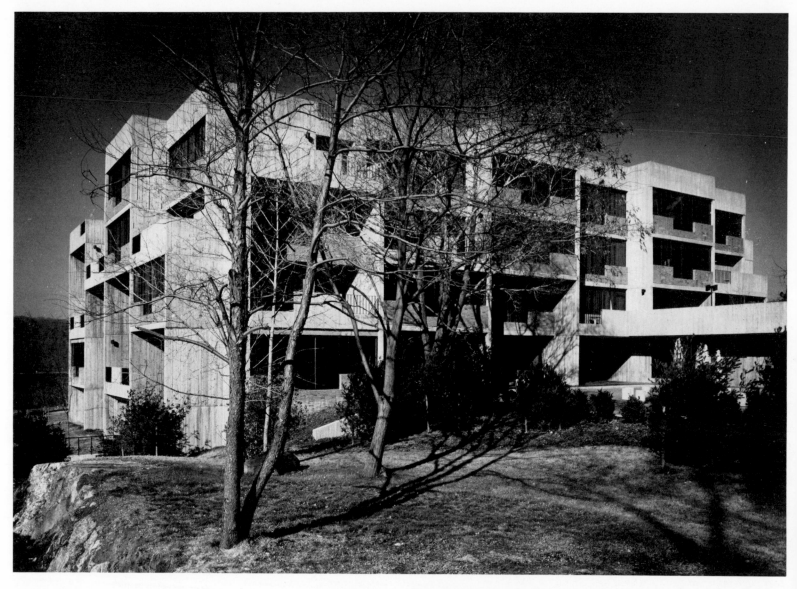

Side view showing the Goldfine Pavillion and the connecting wing to the old building. (*Photographer: Max Gruzen*)

HEBREW HOME FOR THE AGED AT RIVERDALE PALISADE NURSING HOME BRONX, NEW YORK

Site

The Hebrew Home for the Aged at Riverdale, a vital and growing medical-social community, serves more than 800 residents. The latest addition to its building program is an eight-story, 348-bed facility —the Palisade Nursing Home.

The Home, whose focal point is a turn-of-the-century mansion, is on a 19-acre site on the bank of the Hudson River. It is bordered on the east by Palisade Avenue in a scenic residential area of the Bronx and, on the west by the river, about 20 minutes north of midtown Manhattan. Recent additions, designed by Gruzen & Partners, were carefully planned to relate to the unusually dramatic site through a series of walkways, a landscaped terrace and service spaces, which unify the different structures both functionally and visually.

Because of the locations of the two newest residential units—the Goldfine Pavilion, completed in 1968, and the Palisade Nursing Home—1975—many rooms have spectacular views of the Hudson River and New Jersey Palisades. A variety of views compensate for the limited mobility of some of the home's residents, whose average age is currently 82. A one-story service structure between the new residential pavilions provides indoor circulation routes for residents, staff, food and supplies. The roof of this service link provides an outdoor plaza facing the Hudson, with tree-lined stairways, promenade decks, dining and recreational spaces.

Nursing Units

The new pavilion (Palisade Nursing Home) includes a 266-bed, long-term care facility occupying five of the eight floors. Accommodations here include 34 single and 116 double bedrooms. Two floors of this facility also have been designated as health-related residential units, where the environment and services can be tailored to fit the needs of those who may require a level of care between an ambulatory and infirmary unit. Accommodations of this section include 28 single and 27 double bedrooms, each with a separate sitting room, accommodating 82 well-aged residents.

Ancillary Areas

The first floor of the new pavilion offers complete medical and den-

tal services consisting of: physicians' examining and treatment rooms; podiatry and opthamology offices; x-ray department; physical, hydro-, and occupational therapy studios; hematology and urology laboratories; pharmacy; central supply and sterilizaton room; medical records library; and medical, clinical nurse and administration offices. The pavilion also features complete dietary services in a new kitchen, which serves the entire complex; beauty and barber shops; coffee shop/nightclub; and maintenance and housekeeping offices. A large portion of the existing main building was renovated, and the existing kitchen was converted into a special staff dining area.

Construction

Construction of the new pavilion is of steel framing with brick exterior matching that of the existing architecture. It is fully air-conditioned and has a centrally piped oxygen supply with individual bedside outlets and an advanced fire alarm and sprinkler system.

Financing

Financial assistance was provided to the Home by a program similar to the Mitchell-Lama Housing Program (article 28-A under the Housing and Home Finance Agency of the State of New York and administered by the Department of Health).

Project Summary

Owner: Palisade Nursing Home Company, Inc.,
  5901 Palisade Avenue, Bronx, New York 10471
Architect: Gruzen & Partners, Architects-Planners,
  New York, New York
Structural Engineer: Harwood & Gould
Mechanical Engineer: Batlan & Oxman
Landscape Architect: M. Paul Friedberg and Associates
Interior Design Consultant: Bill Bagnall Associates
Food Consultant: Romano-Gatland & Associates
General Contractor: Starrett Brothers and Eken, Inc.
Site: 19 acres
Number of beds: 348
Number of floors: 8

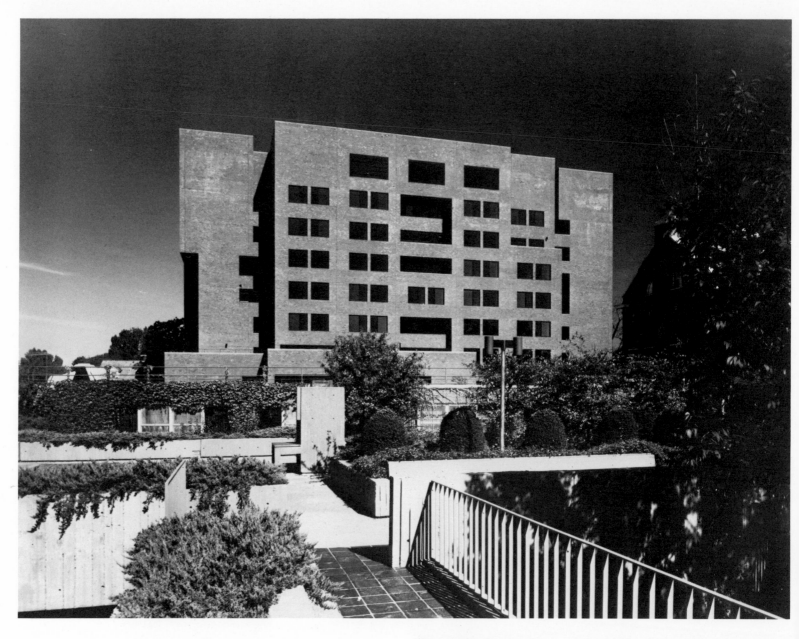

The Palisade Nursing Home, newest addition to the Hebrew Home for the Aged. The new landscaped terrace is seen in the foreground. (*Photographer: Nathaniel Lieberman*)

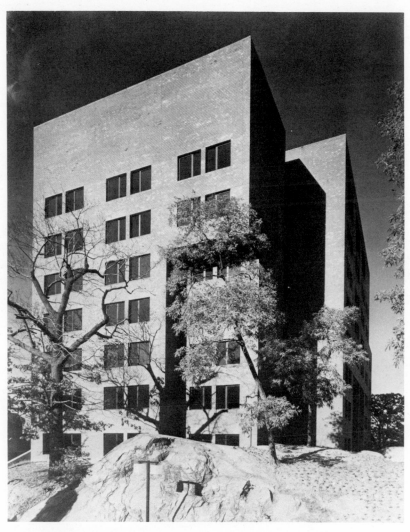

Side view of building and natural rock formations as it has become part of the landscape. (*Photographer: Nathaniel Lieberman*)

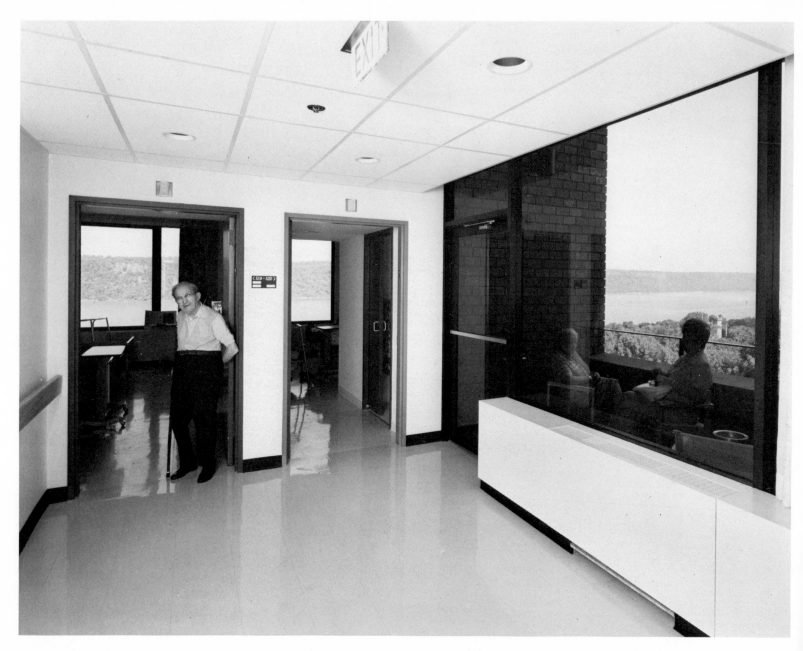

View of corridor and terrace overlooking the Hudson River. (*Photographer: Nathaniel Lieberman*)

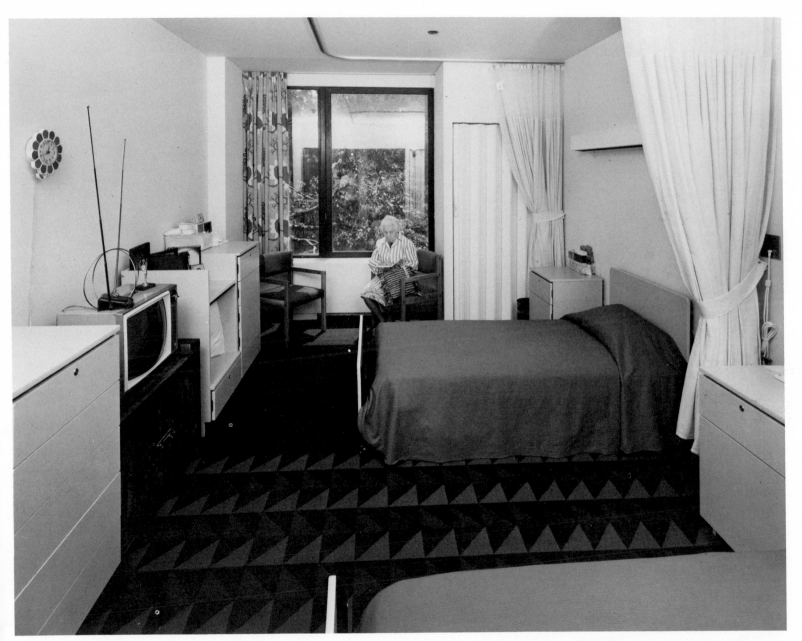

Double bedded room. (*Photographer: Nathaniel Lieberman*)

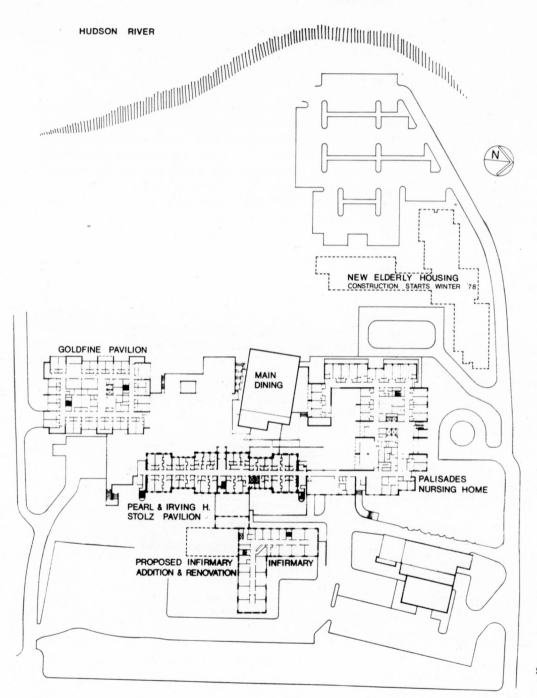

HUDSON RIVER

GOLDFINE PAVILION

MAIN DINING

NEW ELDERLY HOUSING
CONSTRUCTION STARTS WINTER '78

N

PALISADES
NURSING HOME

PEARL & IRVING H.
STOLZ PAVILION

PROPOSED INFIRMARY
ADDITION & RENOVATION   INFIRMARY

**Site plan showing the entire complex.
The Hebrew Home for the Aged at Riverdale.**

DAUGHTERS OF SARAH NURSING HOME
ALBANY, NEW YORK

The daughters of Sarah Nursing Home, located on part of a 50-acre site on the outskirts of Albany, New York, is a 202-bed facility that replaced an outmoded 123-bed home located in Troy, New York. The project was constructed for Daughters of Sarah Nursing Home, Inc., a corporation sponsored by the Daughters of Sarah Jewish Home, Inc., a nonprofit sponsor, under provisions of the Nursing Home Companies Law, Article 28-A, New York State Public Health Law administered by the New York State Department of Health. Construction started in August 1971 and was completed in April 1973, under a Construction Management/General Contractor agreement with Sano-Rubin Construction Company, Inc., of Albany, New York.

Program Requirements

The program requirements were an outgrowth of the sponsor's experience in developing an holistic approach to care of the aged, encompassing advanced medical, social, psychiatric and nursing care services. A basic program objective was the creation of residential "streets," resident "neighborhoods" and a "downtown" central core. Early decisions were made to adhere to the following program:

Single resident rooms only, with private toilet
   facilities for each room
50 resident beds per nursing unit
A one-story plan
A special care unit for treatment of acute illnesses
Shared facilities for nursing stations and resident
   areas to reduce costs
Decentralized sterilization
Short resident corridors

During the early planning, an outpatient day care program serving 50 residents from the community was added and programmed spaces were increased accordingly. Room designs were based on a complete mockup, locating window, heating/cooling unit and plumbing fixtures; this was constructed in the original home during the preliminary design phase.

Construction

The roof system is structural steel with metal deck to provide a one-hour fire rated construction throughout. Exterior walls are panel brick with light colored porcelain enamel panels above and below vinyl covered wood casement windows. Interior partitions are predominately gypsum board on metal studs, with glazed partitions in recreation, dining and lounge areas. All resident and public spaces are air-conditioned, and the entire facility is electrically heated. Each resident room has individual temperature control.

Future Expansion

The facility has been designed for future growth. The addition of a 100-bed patient center, very similar in configuration to the present ones, would complete an internal circulation path while maintaining the same space relationship of the present resident centers to the central core. Only the occupational and physical therapy areas of the core would have to be enlarged to accommodate the additional 100 beds, and initial planning provides for easy expansion of these areas.

Project Summary

Architect: Donald J. Stephens Associates
Structural Engineer: John T. Percy
Mechanical/Electrical Engineer: Robert D. Krouner
Site: 50 acres
Number of Beds: 202
Number of Parking Spaces: 214
Number of Floors: One
Gross Area of Building: 126,700 square feet (including 12,500 square
   feet for day care program)
Gross Area Per Bed: 568 square feet
Number of Beds Per Nursing Station: 50
Proportion of Women to Men Residents: 3:1

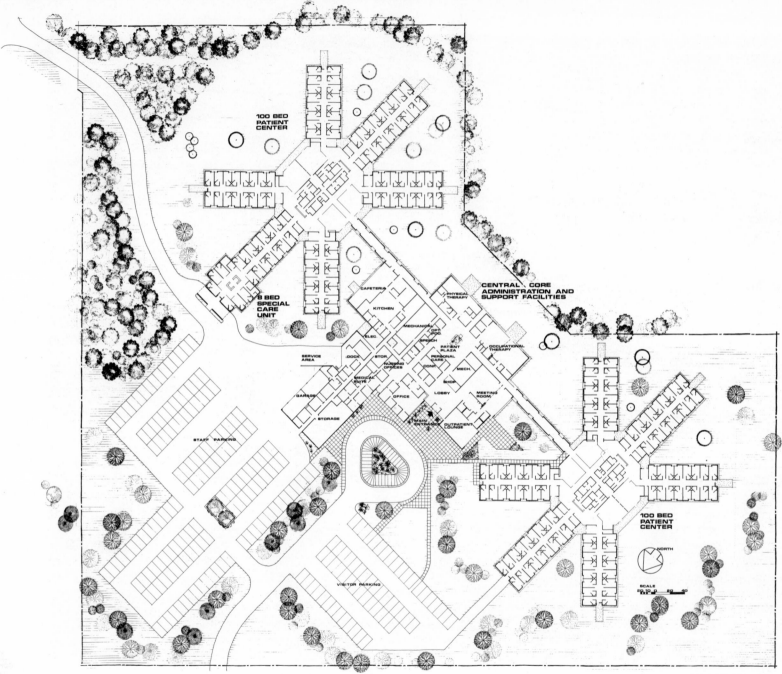

100 BED PATIENT CENTER

8 BED SPECIAL CARE UNIT

CAFETERIA

KITCHEN

MECHANICAL

ELEC.

SERVICE AREA

DOCK

STOR.

NURSING OFFICES

MEDICAL SUITE

GARAGE

OFFICE

STORAGE

MAIN ENTRANCE

PHYSICAL THERAPY

CENTRAL CORE ADMINISTRATION AND SUPPORT FACILITIES

OPT. POD.

SPEECH

PATIENT PLAZA

PERSONAL CARE

CONF.

SHOP

LOBBY

MECH.

OCCUPATIONAL THERAPY

MEETING ROOM

OUTPATIENT LOUNGE

STAFF PARKING

VISITOR PARKING

100 BED PATIENT CENTER

NORTH

SCALE

Overall site plan.

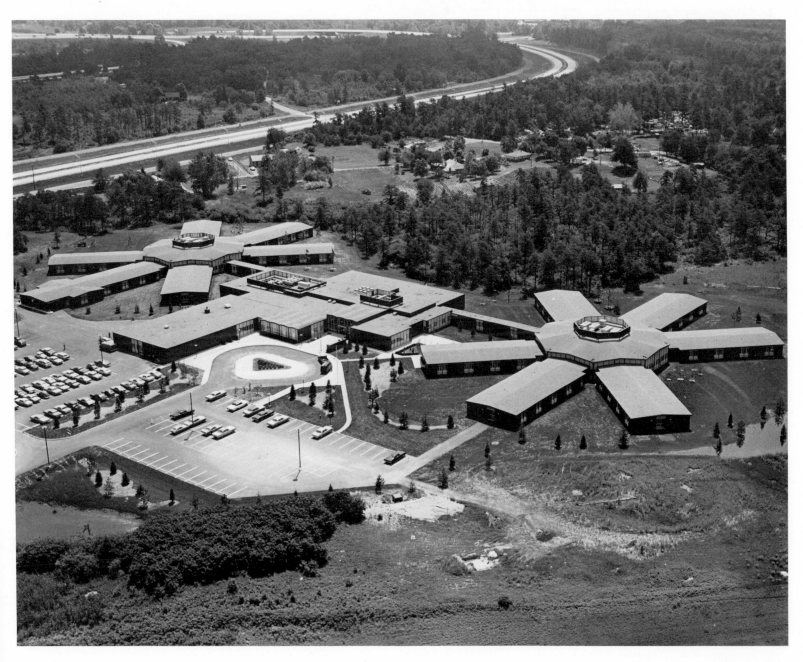

Aerial view of completed project.

175

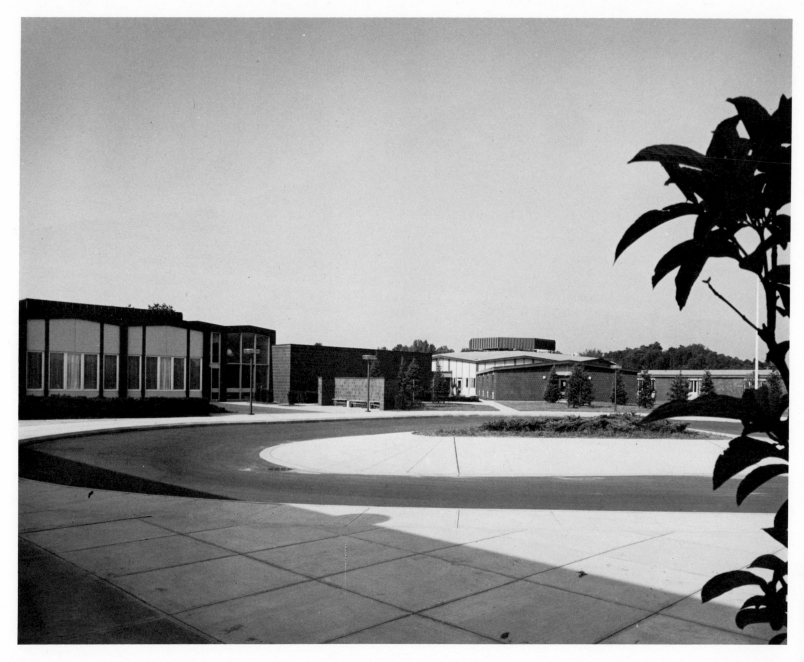

Main entrance.

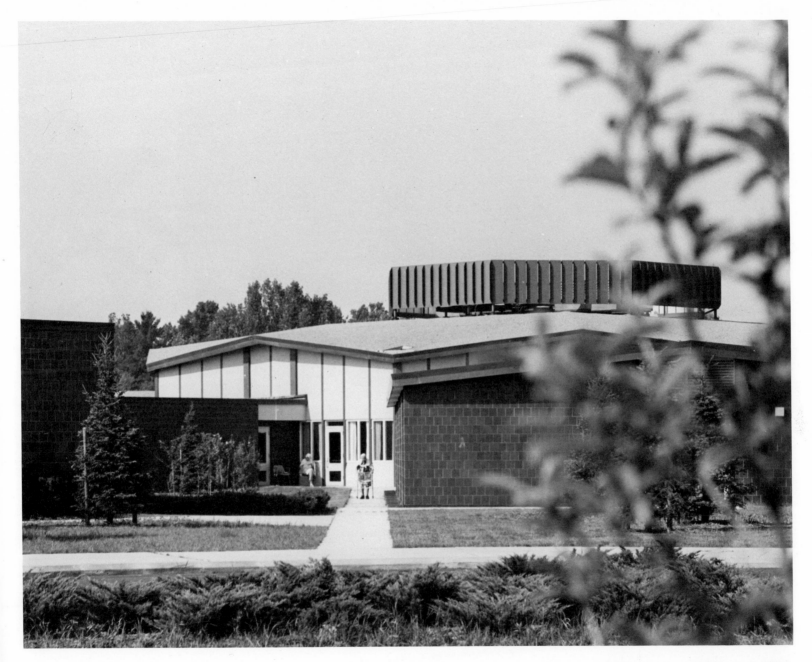

Outdoor area for walking or just sitting.

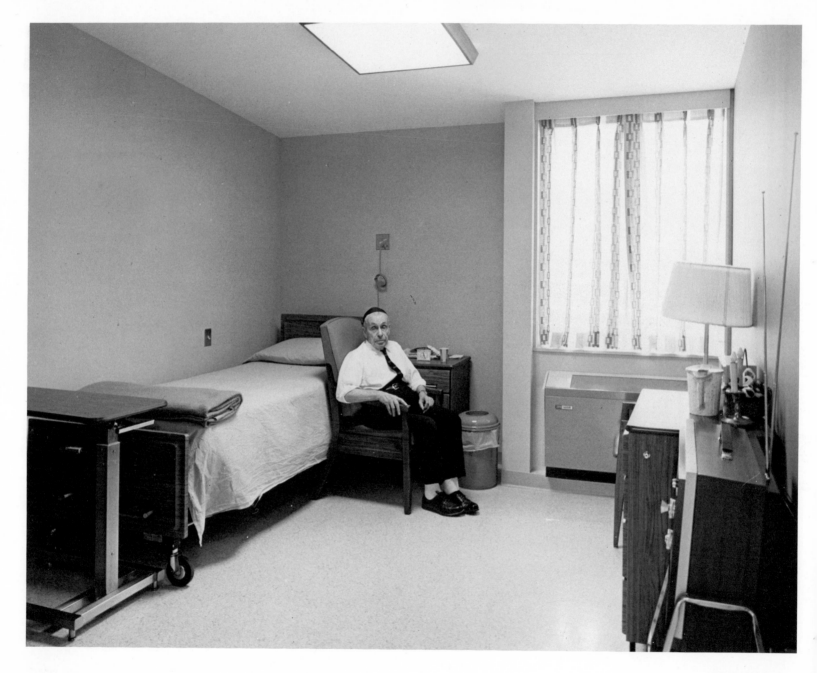

Private bedroom.

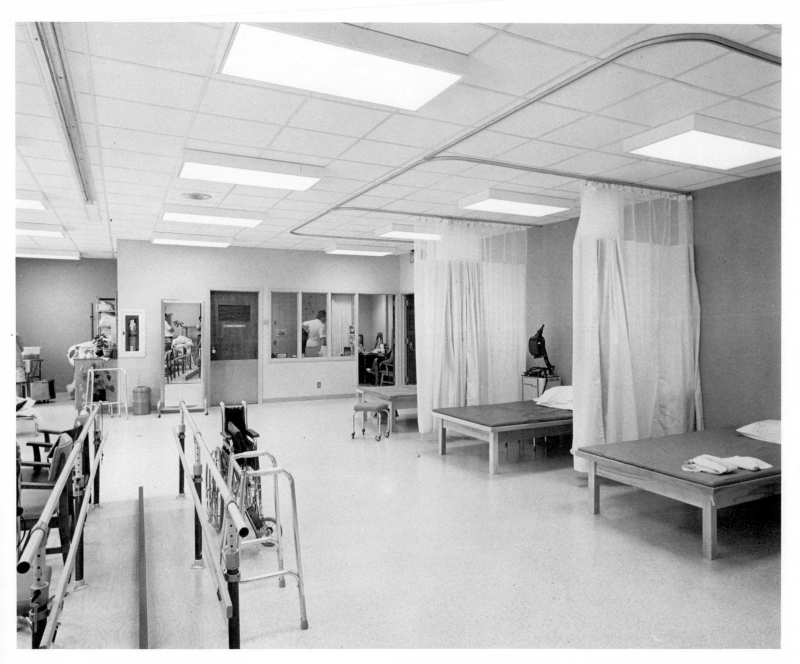

Physical therapy room.

McLEAN HOME, SIMSBURY, CONNECTICUT

Site

The site, with its gently rolling topography and natural woodland areas provides seasonal changes in color that heightens the daily experience and integrates the flowing forms of the structure to it. It is located 10 minutes by bus from the historic town of Simsbury and 20 minutes from Hartford. Various activities in the locality are available. The area provides a rich source of volunteer help. Community participation is a vital adjunct to the residents' well-being. The site is a part of the estate of the late Sen. George Payne McLean, who died in 1932. Sen. McLean provided for the concept of the Home in his will as a memorial to his mother.

The Building Design

As one approaches the entrance, the curvilinear forms welcome the visitor and provide a sense of security and well-being. The materials, concrete, brick and glass, blend quietly with the natural background. Immediately upon entering, there is a sense of warmth and excitement given off by the visual reaction to the design of the central circular mall that links the social areas with adjacent health and residential facilities.

This central area was conceived of as a neighborhood shopping center, with its central fireplace, conversation area, gift shop, library, dining hall, snack bar, game rooms and educational activities. The use of these activities are a vital part of the everyday life of the residents. In addition, it is here that community participation will originate. Artists will exhibit, lecturers, therapists and various commentators will discuss subjects of everyday interest.

Nursing Units

Adjacent to the "Mall" is the residential nursing care wing known as the "Triad," a name developed from the geometric forms of its plan: an equilateral triangle with curved concave sides. The wing is two stories high and contains 120 beds. The residential rooms are on the exterior perimeter and in the center are the rehabilitative and treatment facilities. By virtue of its design, the resident corridors are provided with recessed areas at each bedroom entrance and lounges at various areas. These "places" create an interesting series of activity centers that serve an important social need for those residents who cannot venture too far from their rooms. The interiors are treated in bright colors and lively graphics to assist the need for orientation and to produce a more cheerful environment.

Finally, every resident can enjoy the beauty of the outdoors, either sitting on the terrace or, if completely ambulant, taking advantage of the pleasant nature walks surrounding the building. The exterior design of the terraces and the rooms themselves in the curvilinear plan articulates these areas, so that the residential scale is strengthened. Thus, the total environment achieves a sense of intimate human relationships from within, plus the smooth blending of form with the natural beauty of the exterior.

Residents' Rooms

To attain a residential look, some of the furnishings were custom designed: wardrobe units with adjustable rails, clothing closets, book shelves, pull-out desks and flip-down drawer fronts, which permit viewing the contents from wheelchair level. Each room has a sliding glass door leading to a balcony on the second floor or to a patio on the first floor.

Color

Very strong primary colors are evident everywhere; even the bedroom ceilings are treated with color. One of the residents commented that it was shocking at first, but now they all love the profusion of strong colors. There are three color schemes for resident rooms. The ceilings were painted in different colors to provide bedridden residents with a cheerful overlook. Corridor recesses in the nursing wing were painted alternating bright colors, giving sparkle and life to the room entrances and assisting in orienting and identifying one's room.

Project Summary

Architect: Katz Waisman Weber
Structural Engineer: Pfisterer, Tor and Assoc.
Mechanical/Electrical Engineers: Dubin, Mindell, Bloome Assoc.
Interior Designer: Eve Frankl Interiors and Hans Krieks Associates
Landscape Architect: Allen W. Hixon, Jr.
Builder: Dimeo Construction Co.
Site: 53 acres
Number of beds: 120
Total building area: 87,000 square feet
Area per bed: 725 square feet
Total cost: $3,800,000
Cost per bed: $31,666
Cost per square foot: $43.67

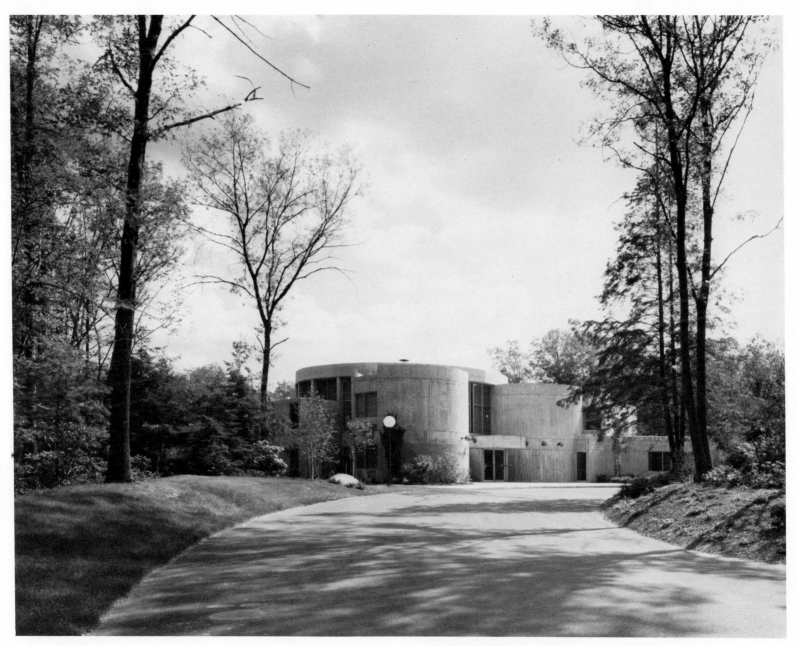

View of main entrance showing exposed, reinforced concrete construction. (*Photographer: Robert Galbraith*)

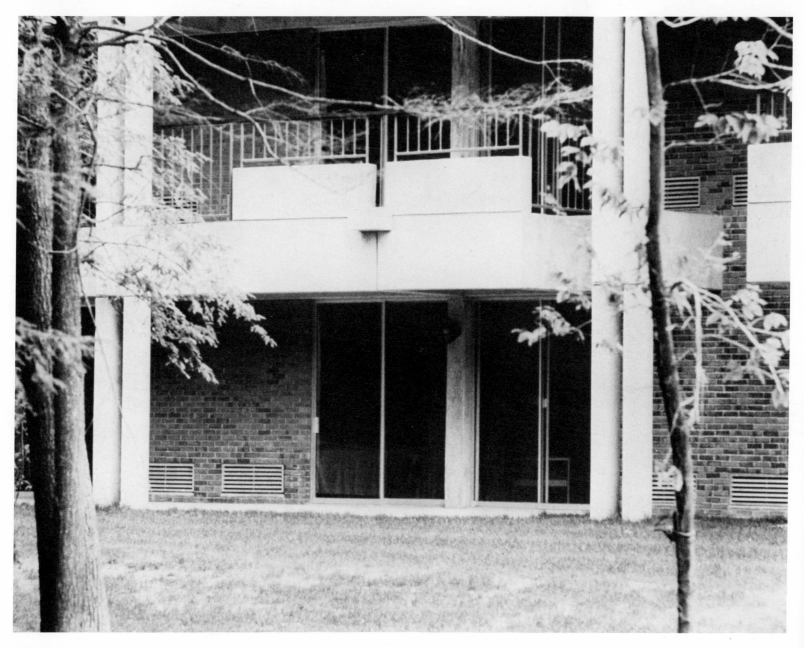

Exterior view of resident rooms. Each room has outdoor access through sliding glass doors. (*Photographer: Robert Galbraith*)

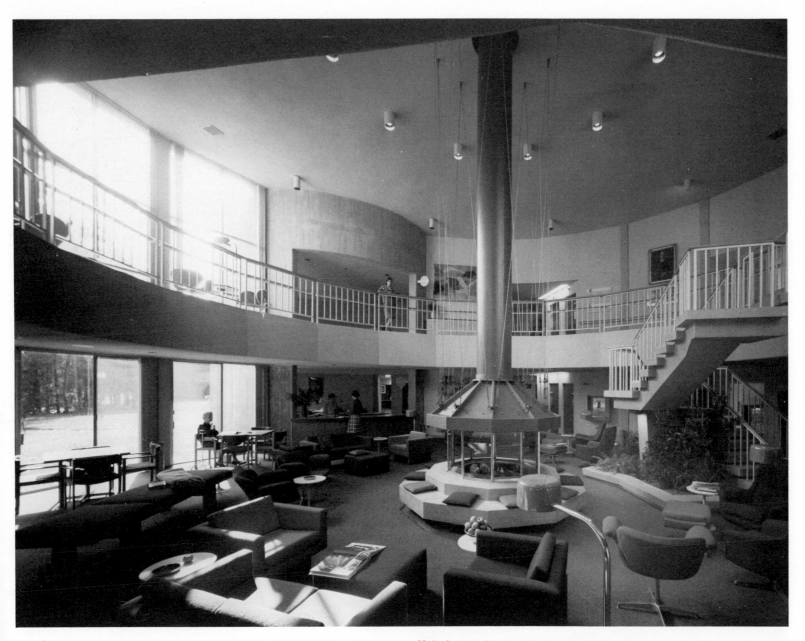

Main lounge is one of several meeting places for residents and guests. Second floor balcony leads to other activity areas. (*Photographer: Robert Galbraith*)

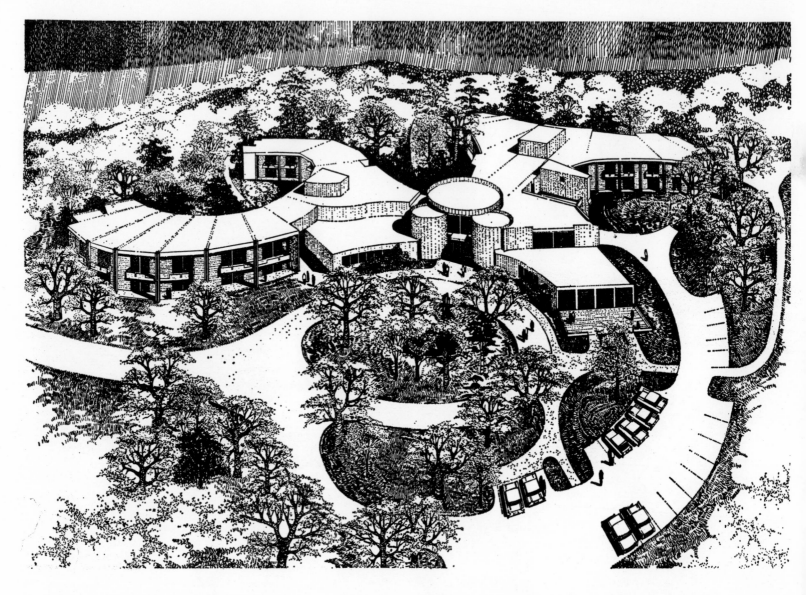

Aerial view of the entire project. To date only about half is completed, containing 120 beds.

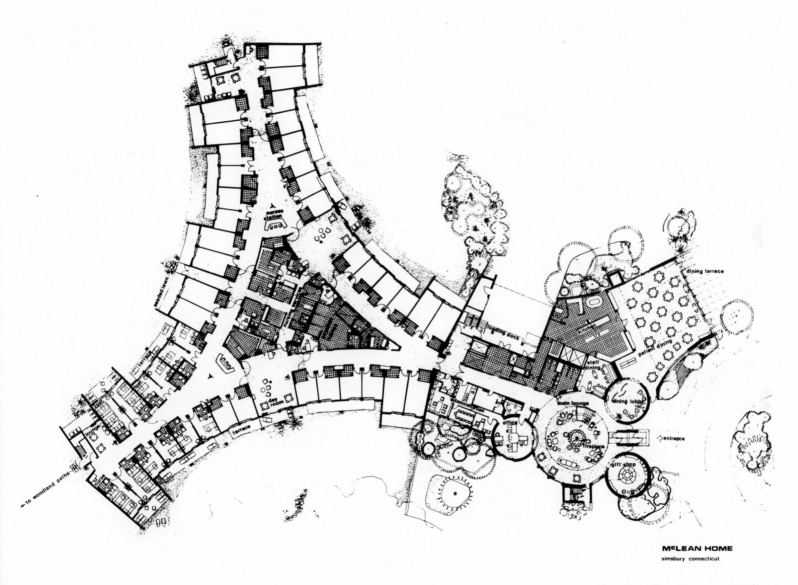

M^cLEAN HOME
simsbury connecticut

First floor plan of the completed part.

MAPLE KNOLL VILLAGE
SPRINGDALE, OHIO

Site

This new community for senior citizens is located on a triangular site in a residential area near Cincinnati, Ohio. An impressive cluster of large trees surrounding a gently rising knoll forms the main feature of the basically flat site. Nearby shopping facilities and major arteries leading to Cincinnati can be reached by a road which adjoins the site.

Program

The program for Maple Knoll Village called for a comprehensive care facility for the aging to consist of: a) an independent living component of 150 apartments; b) an intermediate and skilled nursing unit of 165 beds; c) extensive support, recreational and rehabilitative facilities serving residents and patients; d) various out-reach programs for the elderly, including an adult day-care center; e) a pre-school facility to serve neighborhood children; and f) master planning of the entire site to accommodate a future population of 600 residents.

Solution

Maple Knoll Village provides an environment for the aging which offers meaning and encourages community involvement. It is designed as three linked structures: independent living facility, nursing care unit and shared common facility; all buildings are oriented in an arc around the landscaped knoll and cluster of trees. The knoll, or Village Green, is thus the focal point, enclosed and defined by the buildings of the Village itself. The three buildings are joined by Main Street, an interior circulation spine which serves as the principal gathering and activity center for the residents. Main Street is broad, skylit and connects to all the enclosed activity centers, with lounges, solaria and winter garden at intervals along its path. Major activity spaces, such as dining rooms, workshops and studios, as well as portions of Main Street, face toward the Village Green.

The shared facilities are located between the independent living and nursing care units. These include a winter garden, solarium, chapel, auditorium, beauty and barber shops, gift shop, snack bar, occupational therapy rooms, arts and crafts workshops and administrative offices.

The independent living facility includes 150 efficiency, one-bedroom and two-bedroom apartments. These are served by dining rooms, lounges, club rooms, a library and guest rooms. Space is provided for outdoor dining and courtyards, as well as small private terraces for lower-level apartments.

The nursing care unit contains 116 intermediate care beds and a skilled nursing section of 49 beds. It is served by medical examination rooms, treatment rooms, physical and occupational therapy areas, dental services, dining rooms and recreation and social service spaces. On the main floor is a day-care center for senior citizens and a Montessori-type nursery school, where residents are welcome to participate as volunteers. Access to the Village is from a road system which forms a loop around the rear of the three main buildings. It will serve as a spine for future development. Thirty units of single-story cluster housing have been built across the road near the multi-story independent living facility. Parking is provided in seven landscaped zones for a total of 261 cars.

Construction

The total area of the three main structures is 290,000 square feet. Construction of the independent living and nursing care units is of masonry bearing walls and precast concrete planks. Basement areas and the shared facilities unit are framed with a poured-in-place column and concrete flat slab system. The buildings are faced with an iron spot dark brick. The cluster housing units are of simple wood frame construction with stained cedar siding and asphalt roof shingles. The construction cost was approximately $12,500,000.

Project Summary

Owner: Southwestern Ohio Seniors' Services, Inc.,
   11100 Springfield Pike, Springdale, Ohio 45246
Architect: Gruzen & Partners, New York, New York
Associate Architect: Glaser & Meyers and Associates, Inc.
   Cincinnati, Ohio
Structural Engineer: Robert Silman Associates
Mechanical Engineer: Syska & Hennessy, Inc.
Landscape Architect: M. Paul Friedberg and Associates
Food Service Consultant: Romano/Gatland
Construction Manager: Gruzen/Amis

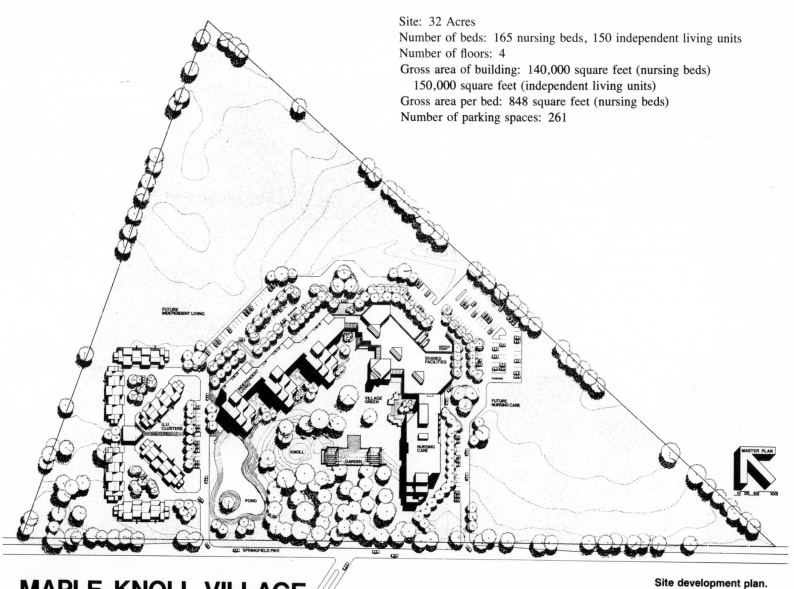

Site: 32 Acres
Number of beds: 165 nursing beds, 150 independent living units
Number of floors: 4
Gross area of building: 140,000 square feet (nursing beds)
   150,000 square feet (independent living units)
Gross area per bed: 848 square feet (nursing beds)
Number of parking spaces: 261

Site development plan.

MAPLE KNOLL VILLAGE

SPRINGDALE OHIO /   A HOME FOR THE AGING
FOR THE SOUTHWESTERN OHIO SENIORS' SERVICES, INC

GRUZEN & PARTNERS
ARCHITECTS PLANNERS ENGINEERS
1700 BROADWAY NEW YORK . N.Y. 10019

GLASER & MYERS AND ASSOC. INC
ASSOCIATE ARCHITECTS
2753 ERIE AVENUE CINCINNATI, OHIO 45208

MECHANICAL ENGINEER
BYBKA & HENNESBY, INC. ENGR.
FOOD SERVICE CONSULTANT
ROMANO AND ASSOCIATES

LANDSCAPE ARCHITECTS
M. PAUL FRIEDBERG ASSOC.
STRUCTURAL ENGINEERS
ZOLDOS/BILMAN CONSULT. ENGR.

DATE

JOB NUMBER
1165

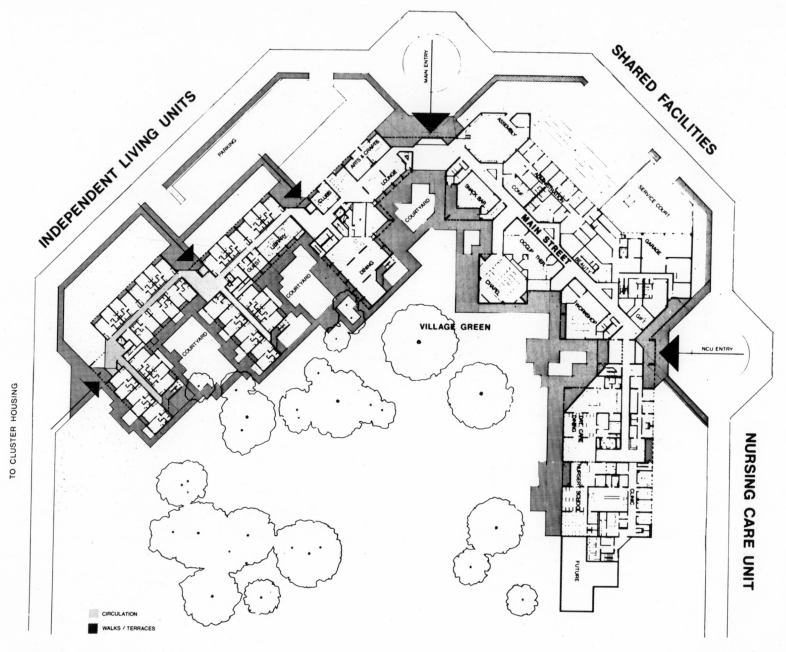

INDEPENDENT LIVING UNITS

SHARED FACILITIES

NURSING CARE UNIT

TO CLUSTER HOUSING

MAIN ENTRY

PARKING

ARTS & CRAFTS

LOUNGE

CLUBS

COURTYARD

LIBRARY

GUEST

DINING

COURTYARD

COURTYARD

SNACK BAR

CONF

ADMINISTRATION

MAIN STREET

BEAUTY

ASSEMBLY

SERVICE COURT

GARAGE

OCCUP. THER.

CHAPEL

WORKSHOP

GIFT

VILLAGE GREEN

NCU ENTRY

DAY CARE

DINING

NURSERY SCHOOL

CLINIC

FUTURE

CIRCULATION

WALKS / TERRACES

Main floor plan.

188

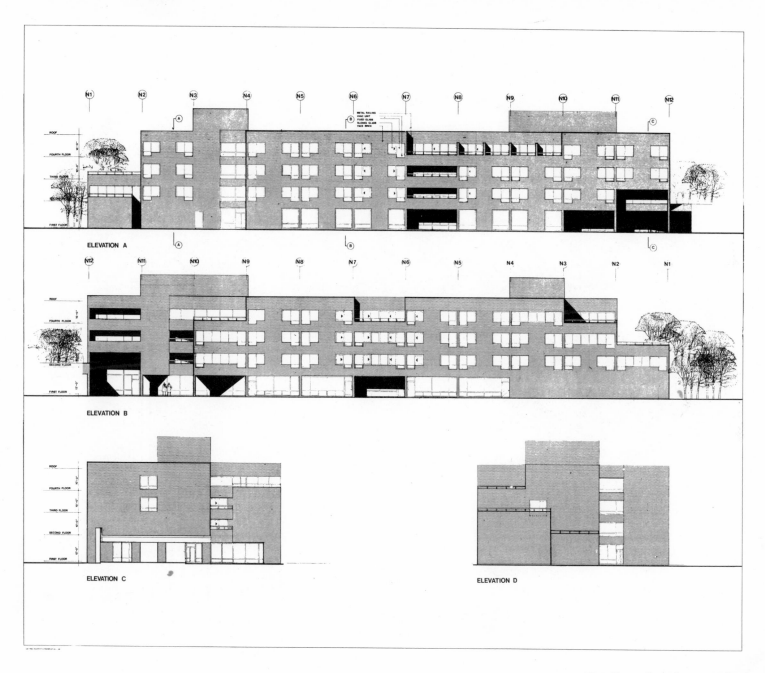

ELEVATION A

ELEVATION B

ELEVATION C

ELEVATION D

Elevations of nursing care wing.

189

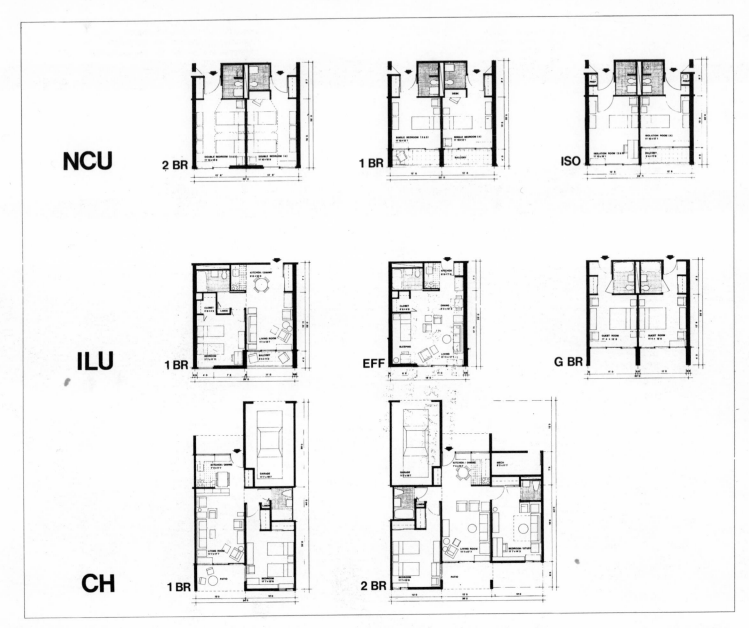

NCU

2 BR   1 BR   ISO

ILU

1 BR   EFF   G BR

CH

1 BR   2 BR

Typical unit plans.

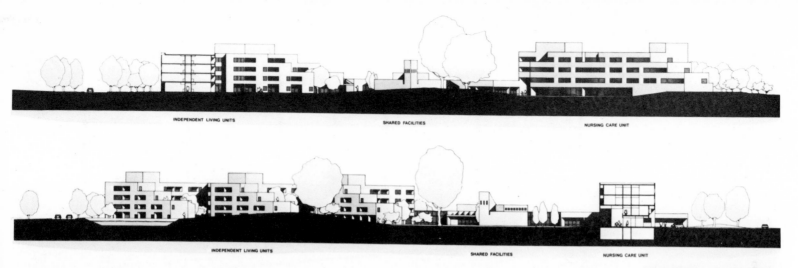

INDEPENDENT LIVING UNITS

SHARED FACILITIES

NURSING CARE UNIT

INDEPENDENT LIVING UNITS

SHARED FACILITIES

NURSING CARE UNIT

Elevations of Village Green.

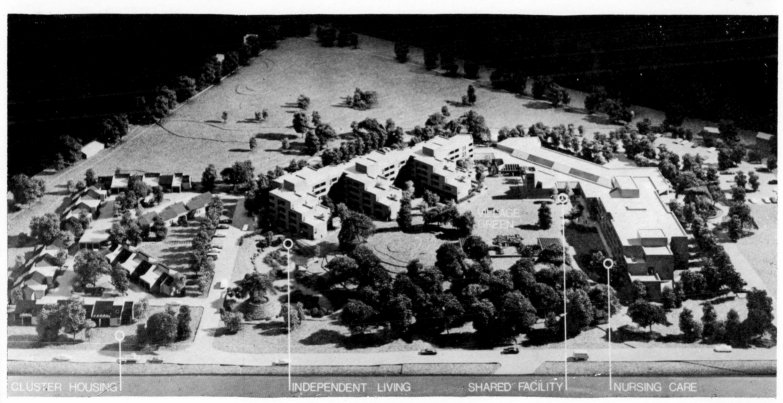

VILLAGE GREEN

CLUSTER HOUSING

INDEPENDENT LIVING

SHARED FACILITY

NURSING CARE

Model photo.

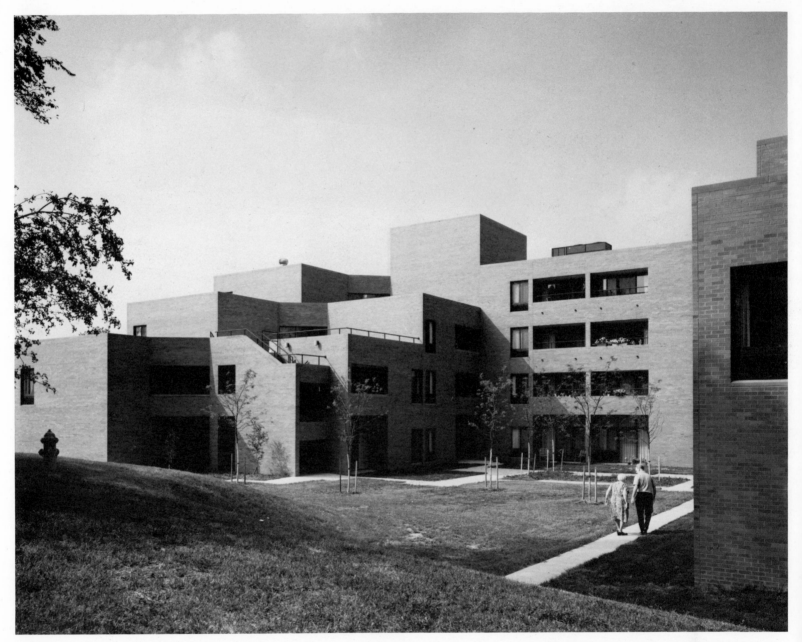

Exterior view of building (*Photographer: Bo Parker*).

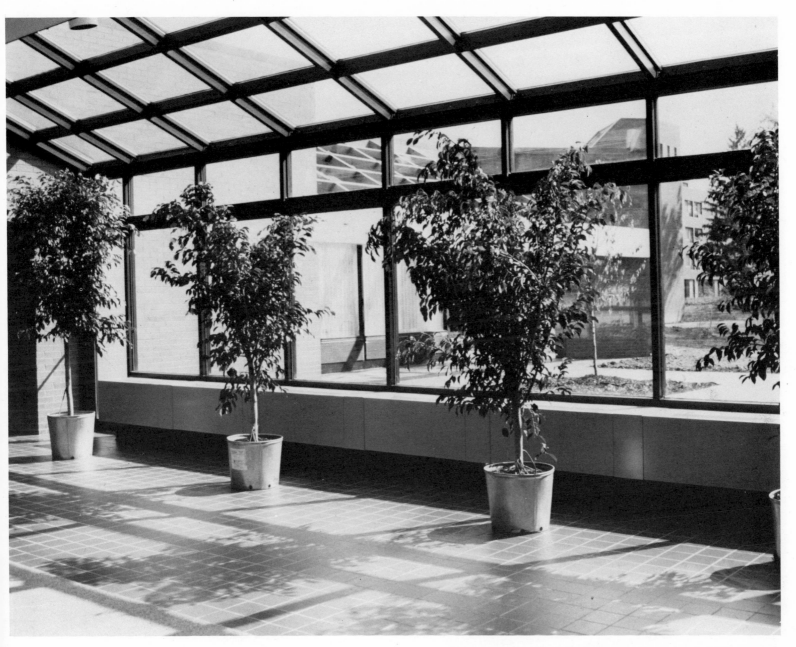

Glass enclosed portion of "Main Street" (*Photographer: Bo Parker*).

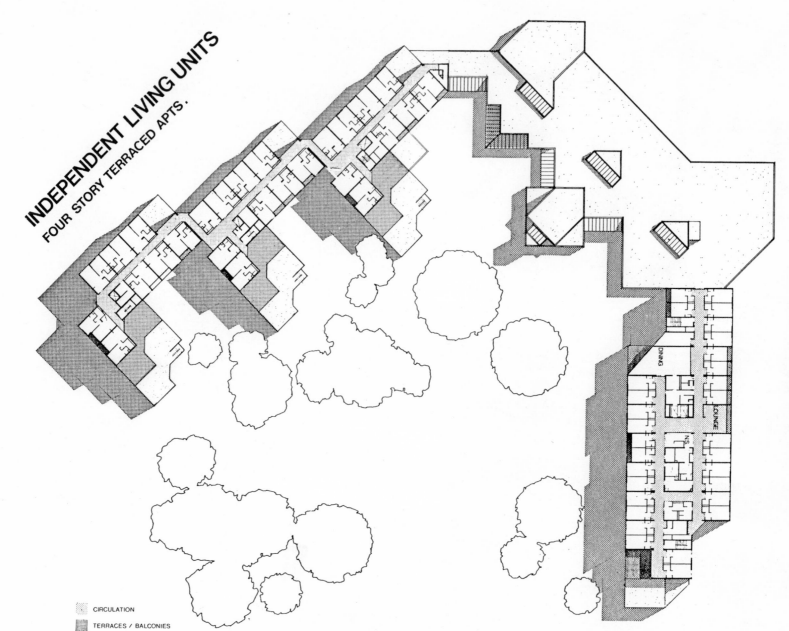

INDEPENDENT LIVING UNITS

FOUR STORY TERRACED APTS.

NURSING CARE UNITS

DINING

LOUNGE

NS

CIRCULATION

TERRACES / BALCONIES

Typical floor plan.

194

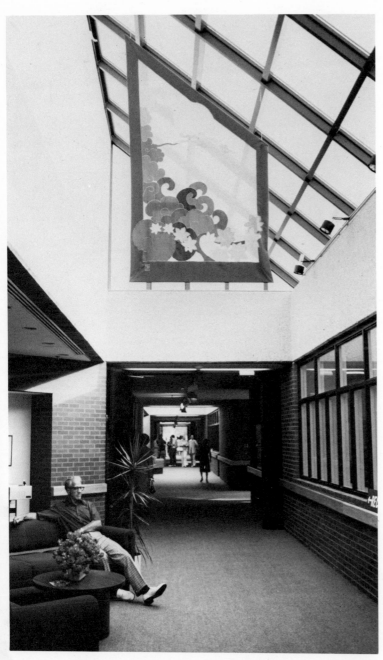

Sitting areas along "Main Street" (*Photographer: Bo Parker*).

JEWISH INSTITUTE FOR GERIATRIC CARE
NEW HYDE PARK, LONG ISLAND, NEW YORK

This building is located within a medical center campus, and it is an integral part of this important urban complex. The geriatric resident receives total medical, surgical, psychiatric and rehabilitative services. The architects developed three levels of duplex residential units with indoor and outdoor porches at each level. On the interior, these units are planned to house six residents, whose rooms are clustered about a "front porch" which opens to the main corridor or "street." During the summer months, the residents can sit outside on the "back porches."

By virtue of this design concept the residents are encouraged to socialize in small groups. The plan is designed so that a resident will meet with one group on the front porch and a different group on the back porch, naturally increasing the resident's circle of friends. The back porches are designed to have every other porch set back in the vertical plane; this allows for conversation between neighbors on different floors. In actual practice, the "front porch" idea did not work out as well as anticipated: some residents prefer to see more activity; others are too shy to sit out there.

The section drawing illustrates the basic concept of the project. The residential units are situated on the upper floors above the clinical services, laboratories and out-patient day care center which are located on the second floor. The main entrance level houses the administration, physical and medical rehabilitative unit and the arts and crafts studio. The lower terrace level provides an outdoor garden plaza adjacent to the dining rooms, kitchen and sheltered workshop. All of the major service, storage and mechanical areas are located on this lower level. A connecting tunnel to the full service general hospital allows for the immediate transport of the resident in case of emergency.

Type of Construction

Construction is reinforced concrete. The upper residential floors are arranged as bearing wall boxes; the boxes are supported on the deep, coffered slab located at the third floor level which transfers the load to the concrete columns below. The major finish material of the building is exposed concrete. The exterior has both poured-in-place concrete and pre-cast panels. Clear glass windows and sliding doors are double-glazed. Glass block exterior walls are used at the offices and dining

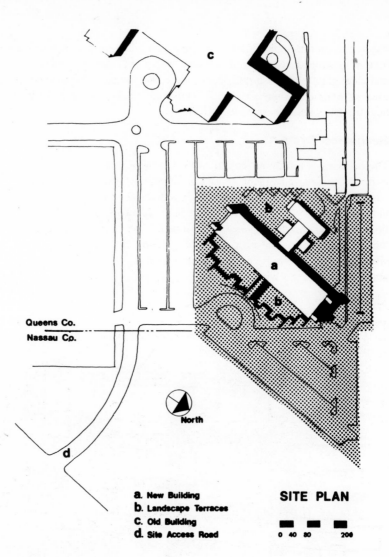

Queens Co.
Nassau Co.

North

a. New Building
b. Landscape Terraces
c. Old Building
d. Site Access Road

SITE PLAN

0 40 80   200

rooms and on the upper floors at the residents' day-dining rooms. The interior partitions are painted gypsum wallboard, fire-proofed wood and clear glass block. Carpet, resilient tile and paving brick have been used as floor covering. Ceiling finishes consist of suspended acoustical tile and exposed concrete coffers.

Mechanical System

The building is totally air conditioned. On the lower three floors, administration areas, resident areas and laboratory areas are separately zoned and controlled. All resident rooms in the top six floors are individually controlled. Most of the residents cannot tolerate air conditioning in the summer, except on extremely hot days. The design of the building reflects the need for resident comfort by reducing excessive heat load demands in summer and allowing solar penetration to assist heating in the winter.

Lighting

In general, lighting is fluorescent, while incandescent fixtures are used in certain areas to change the environmental outlook; i.e., day-

dining rooms, lounges, circulation areas and conference rooms. However, many of the incandescent fixtures are not used because of the high energy requirement and high cost.

Project Summary

Architect: Katz Waisman Weber
Structural Engineer: Lev Zetlin Associates
Mechanical Engineer: Jack Stone, Engineers
Interior Designer: Luss-Kaplan
Landscape Architect: William T. Schmidt
Number of floors: 7
Number of beds: 527
Total building area: 350,000 square feet
Area per bed: 664 square feet
Total cost: $17,600,000
Cost per bed: $33,396.00
Cost per square foot: $50.28
Date of completion: 1973

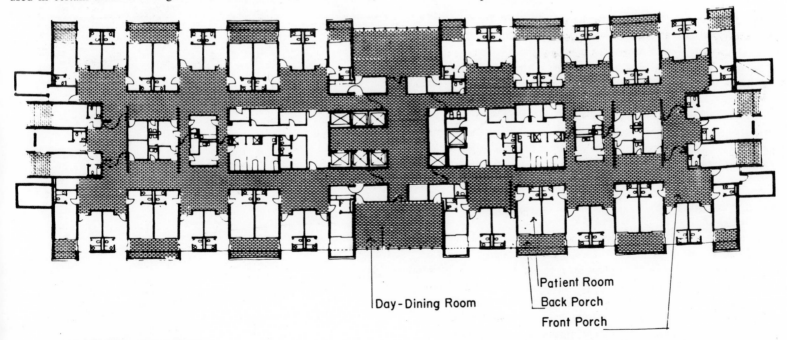

Day-Dining Room

Patient Room

Back Porch

Front Porch

TYPICAL FLOOR

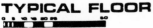

Typical floor plan. Two double and two single rooms form a cluster.

197

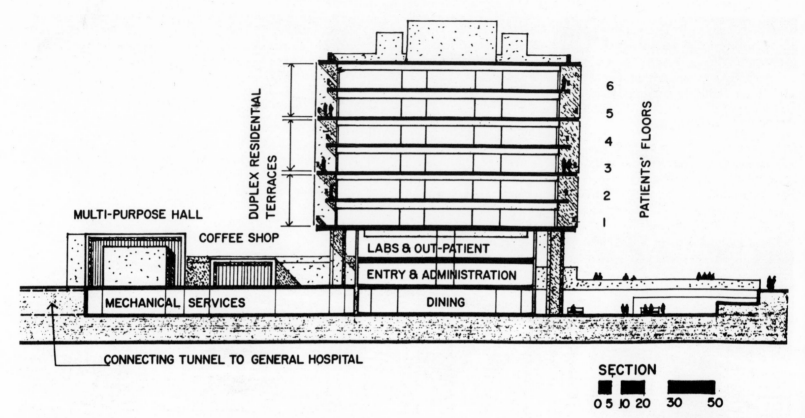

MULTI-PURPOSE HALL

COFFEE SHOP

DUPLEX RESIDENTIAL TERRACES

LABS & OUT-PATIENT

ENTRY & ADMINISTRATION

MECHANICAL SERVICES

DINING

6
5
4
3
2
1

PATIENTS' FLOORS

CONNECTING TUNNEL TO GENERAL HOSPITAL

SECTION

0 5 10 20   30   50

Section through the building.

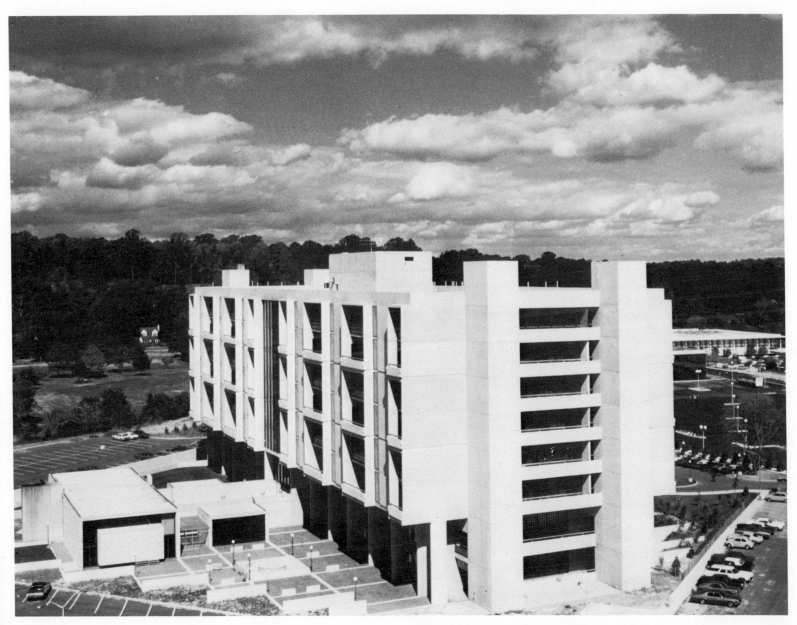

Rear view of the building showing the single story coffee shop and multi-purpose wing. (*Photographer: Robert Galbraith*)

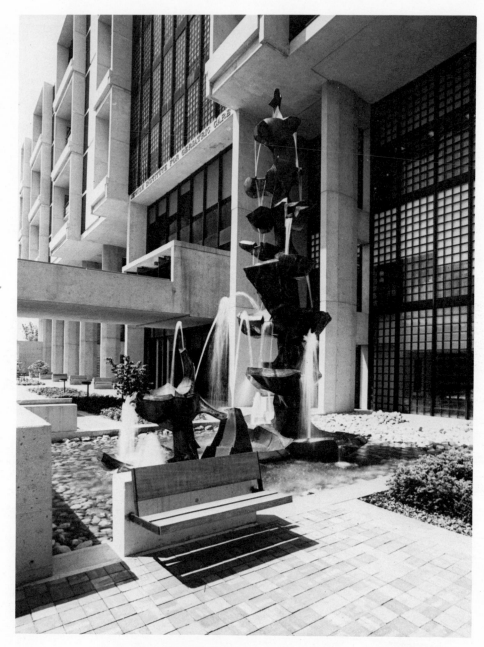

Front view of building showing entrance bridge and landscaped terrace with fountain. (*Photographer: Robert Galbraith*)

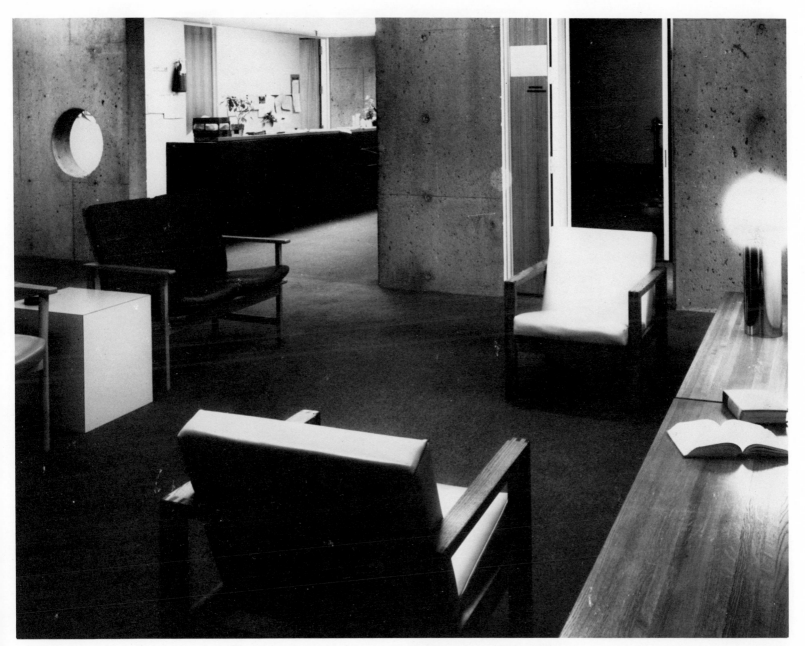

View from residents' day room toward nurses' station. (*Photographer: Robert Galbraith*)

BETH SHOLOM HOME OF EASTERN VIRGINIA
VIRGINIA BEACH, VIRGINIA

This new facility will be part of a statewide system of care for the Jewish elderly in Virginia. After many years of preparatory work, the building was scheduled to be started in 1978, with a completion date scheduled in 1980. The building committee and the architect have visited many fine, long-term care facilities on the East Coast to gain firsthand knowledge of the newest developments in this field. Some of the homes visited are included in this book. As a matter of fact, many of the ideas collected in this book have been used in the design of this building.

Site

The site is just under 10 acres and has some room for future expansion of the nursing facility and for other kinds of housing for the elderly. It is located between a new shopping center and a residential area near major road systems.

Design Considerations

It was decided to limit the number of residents at each nurse's station to forty and the corridors were to be made as short as possible. In addition, the nurse's station would have ample room around it for organized activities, as well as just sitting and "watching the world go by." This basic requirement dictated the eventual layout, which puts the resident rooms on the perimeter and in turn makes the core almost windowless. This will be good for energy conservation, but it may have an adverse effect on the staff and residents. For this reason there will be skylights scattered around the building to bring in natural light.

Recreating the City

There is a small shopping arcade next to the lobby to suggest "downtown," while the nurses' stations will be developed as neighborhoods. The corridors will be named after local streets, providing the residents with a "street address" rather than just a room number. The walls of the corridors leading to the resident rooms will be decorated with supergraphics suggesting building exteriors.

Orientation

There was a great concern for orientation of the residents and the staff within the building. The following steps will be taken to overcome this problem:

- Each neighborhood (nurses' station) will have a different color scheme (orange, yellow and blue).
- The designated color will occur in the floor covering and wall decoration of the corridors leading to the neighborhood.
- Each corridor segment leading to resident rooms will have a different lighting pattern, different ceiling tile pattern and different color scheme.
- Each neighborhood will have different types of lighting fixtures creating markedly different atmosphere.

Construction

- Structural system: steel stud bearing walls and steel joist framed roof.
- Ceiling: suspended acoustical lay-in panels in various sizes and patterns.
- Interior partitions: steel studs and gypsum wallboard.
- Exterior walls: synthetic stucco
- Windows: casement wood with insulating glass.

Project Summary

Architect: The Design Collaborative, Virginia Beach, Va., Laszlo Aranyi, AIA, principal in charge
Structural Engineer: Stroud Engineering Company
Mechanical/Electrical Engineer: Old Dominion Engineering
Construction Manager: R. D. Lambert & Son, Inc.
Interior Designer: Margaret Allen
Site: 9.6 acres
Number of Beds: 120
Number of Floors: 1
Number of Parking Spaces: 66
Gross Area of Building: 61,000 square feet
Gross Area per Bed: 536 square feet
Number of Beds per Nurses Station: 40

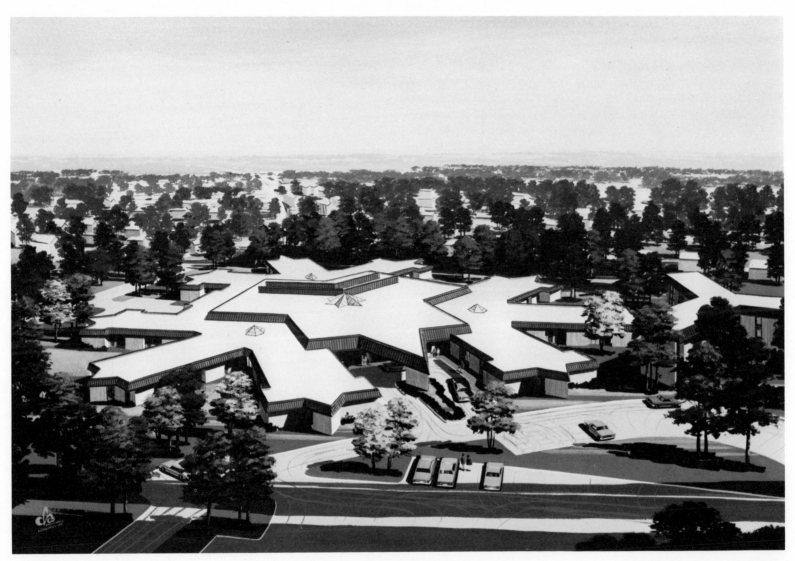

Rendering of proposed building.

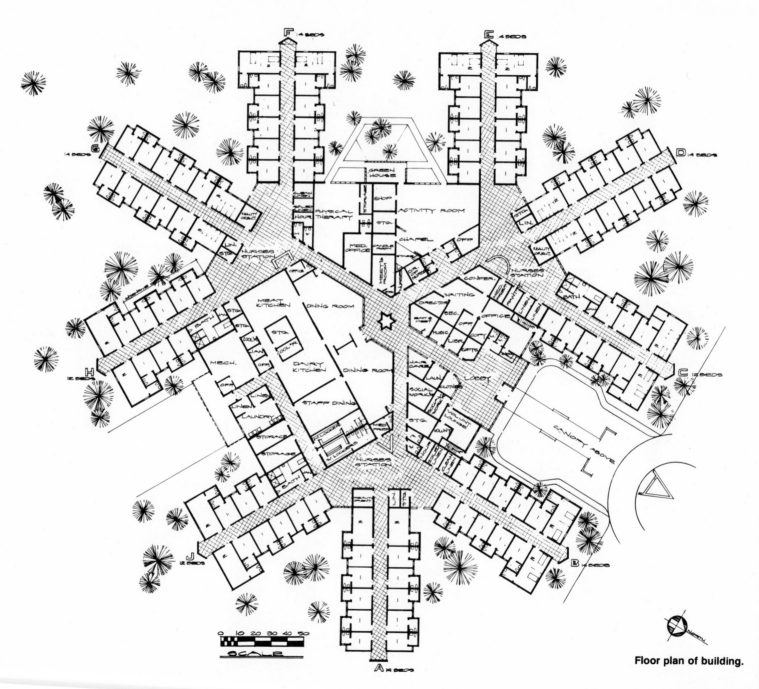

Floor plan of building.

204

SUMMARY OF CASE STUDIES

	Menorah Park	Hebrew Home at Riverdale Goldfine Pavillion	Palisade Nursing Home	Daughters of Sarah	McLean Home	Maple Knoll	Jewish Institute	Beth Sholom
Number of beds:	281	140	348	202	120	165 nursing 150 well-aged	527	120
Total square feet:	189,500	80,000		114,500	87,000	140,000	350,000	61,000
Square feet per bed:	675	571		568	725	848	664	536
Number of single rooms:	147	60	62	202		21	121	84
Size of single rooms:	14 × 14	12 × 14		12 × 12	12 × 12	12 × 12		12 × 12
Number of double rooms:	62	40	143			72	203	18
Size of double rooms:	14 × 18				12 ×19	12 × 15½		12 × 20
Number of beds per nursing station:	24 to 36	40		50	30	55+		40
Number of floors:	2	5	8	1	2	4	7	1
Floor finishes:	Resilient tile	Resilient tile; carpet	Resilient tile; carpet	Resilient tile	Carpet	Resilient tile; carpet	Resilient tile; carpet	Resilient tile; carpet
Wall finishes:		Vinyl wall covering; paint	Vinyl wall covering; paint	Vinyl wall covering	Exposed concrete; painted walls	Vinyl wall covering; painted wallboard	Concrete; brick; painted wallboard	Painted wallboard
Ceiling finishes:	Plaster	Acoustical tile	Acoustical tile	Acoustical tile	Acoustical tile	Acoustical tile; textured paint	Acoustical tile; concrete	Acoustical tile
Heating/air conditioning:	Central	Central	Central	Individual	Individual	Central	Central	Central
Temperature control in resident room:	Yes	Yes	Yes	Yes	Yes	Yes	Yes	Yes
Window types:		Double glazed aluminum	Double gl. alum.	Vinyl covered wood	Aluminum sliding doors	Double glazed; alum.; sliding	Double glazed	Double glazed wood
Structural system:	Concrete	Concrete	Steel	Steel	Concrete	Masonry bearing walls & precast concrete	Concrete	Steel stud bearing & steel
Lighting:	Fluorescent	Fluorescent	Fluorescent	Fluorescent	Fluorescent	Fluorescent Incandescent	Fluorescent Incandescent	Fluorescent Merc. Vapor
Laundry for personal items:		Yes	No	Yes	Yes	Yes		Yes

SUMMARY OF CASE STUDIES

	Menorah Park	Hebrew Home at Riverdale Goldfine Pavillion	Palisade Nursing Home	Daughters of Sarah	McLean Home	Maple Knoll	Jewish Institute	Beth Sholom
Personalization of rooms allowed:	Some	Some	Some	Some	Some	Some	Some	Some
Sheltered workshop:	Yes	Yes	Yes	No	No	Yes	Yes	No
Day care:	Yes		Yes	Yes	No	Yes	No	No
Use of color for orientation:	No	Yes	Yes	Yes	No	Yes	No	Yes
Number of parking spaces:	230			214		261		66
Type of financing:			State	State	Private endowment	Private bond issue	State	Industrial bond
Total cost in millions:	6.4	3.2	12	6.0	3.8	12.5	17.6	3.0
Cost per bed:	22,775	22,857	34,482	29,703	31,666	39,682	33,396	25,000
Date of completion:	1968	1969	1974	1973	1971	1977	1973	1980
Number of employees:	200			306	100		650	

-30-

BIBLIOGRAPHY

The following publications were useful in the preparation of this book and will broaden the reader's understanding of the subject.

1. Doelle, Leslie L.: *Environmental Acoustics*. New York: McGraw-Hill Book Co., 1972.

2. Institutional Management, The News Magazine for Operational Management of Health Care Lodging and Education Facilities, 401 North Broad Street, Philadelphia, Pennsylvania 19108.

3. Koncelik, Joseph A.: *Designing the Open Nursing Home*. PA.: Dowden, Hutchinson and Ross, Inc., 1976.

4. Michigan State Housing Development Authority: *Security Guidelines*. Lansing, Michigan, 1975.

5. Pastalan, Leon A.; Mautz, R. K.; and Merrill, J.: *The Simulation of Age Related Sensory Losses: A New Approach to the Study of Environmental Barriers*. Environmental Design Research, Vol. 1, 1973, p. 383.

6. Public Health Service, Division of Medical Care Administration: *Nursing Homes–Environmental Health Factors*. U.S. Department of Health, Education and Welfare. Publication Number 1009, 1967.

7. Public Health Service, Office of Nursing Home Affairs: *Long-Term Care Facility Improvement Study*. U.S. Department of Health, Education and Welfare. Publication Number (0S)76-50021, July 1975.

8. Research Center, College of Architecture and Environmental Design: *Environmental Criteria: MR Preschool Day Care Facilities*. College Station, Texas: Texas A & M University, 1971.

9. U. S. Department of Commerce, 1976 Survey of Institutionalized Persons: A Study of Persons Receiving Long Term Care. Special Studies Series P-23, No. 69, Issued June 1978.

10. U. S. Department of Housing and Urban Development: *Minimum Property Standards for Care Type Housing*. Publication Number 4920.1

11. Snyder, Lorraine Hiatt and Ostrander, Edward R.: *Research Basis for Behavioral Program, The New York State Veterans' Home, Oxford, New York, New York*. Ithaca: New York State College of Human Ecology, Cornell University, 1974.

12. Snyder, Lorraine Hiatt; Ostrander, Edward R.; and Koncelik, Joseph A., Editors. *The New Nursing Home · Conference Proceedings*. Ithaca: Department of Design and Environmental Analysis, Cornell University, June 1973.

INDEX